Just a Little Run Around the World

ROSIE SWALE POPE

Just a Little Run Around the World

5 years,
3 packs of wolves and
53 pairs of shoes

harper
true

HarperTrue
HarperCollins*Publishers*
77–85 Fulham Palace Road,
Hammersmith, London W6 8JB

www.harpercollins.co.uk

First published by HarperCollins*Publishers* 2009

1

A CIP catalogue record for this book
is available from the British Library

ISBN 978-0-00-730620-6

Printed and bound in Great Britain by
Clays Ltd, St Ives plc

PICTURE CREDITS: Page 1, tl © Rosie Swale Pope, tr © Western Telegraph,
c © Runner's World Images, b © Runner's World Images; page 2, all © Rosie Swale
Pope; page 3, tr & b © Bob Collins, cr © Rosie Swale Pope; page 4, t & cr © Rosie Swale
Pope, cl © Bob Collins, b © Runner's World Images; page 5, t & cr © Rosie Swale Pope;
page 6, tl & cr © Rosie Swale Pope, tr © Karen Christie, bl © Grace Neilsen,
br © Thorgeir Gunnarsson; page 7, t © Thorgeir Gunnarsson, uc © Christine Nielsen;
page 8, t © Malcolm Richards, c © John Pilkington, bl © Rosie Swale Pope,
br © Catherine Addison.

Every effort has been made to trace the owners of copyright material produced herein.
The publishers would like to apologise for any omissions and will be pleased to
incorporate missing acknowledgements in any future editions.

'Things last for ever,
not in years,
but in the moments
in which they happen.'
– *Rosie Swale Pope*

*For Clive,
Eve and James, Pete,
Jayne and Nigel
and the rest of my family
far and wide.*

Author's notes

1. All temperatures are in Celsius (Centigrade) unless otherwise stated.
2. Because of the nature of my route, distances are approximate.

Prologue

Siberia, January 2005

There are a hundred different types of silence in Siberia. The atmosphere becomes part of you. You can sometimes see bare white silver birches in the depth of winter hung with stars on a clear night. In the mesmerising vast forests, dusk in January begins at 2 pm. By then everything is in its hole or nest – or nearly everything.

On a cold, still night, I pull my cart that doubles as a sled, deep into the forest and find some smooth snow among the trees. I put up the tent, collect a bowl of fresh snow to take inside with me to melt on the tiny primus stove for drinks and cooking; it's the nearest thing I have to a kitchen. I have even gathered some icy tree bark from the fallen branches to make tea. The Siberian people have taught me this. It's not quite PG Tips but it's nourishing and tastes fine. Need is a great teacher. I also boil up a few handfuls of buckwheat grain to make a kind of porridge. It's a measure of the power of the silence that even a light footstep outside can make your heart stop. Something is out there.

The night birds – maybe they are jays – suddenly start screeching and chattering. Alert. Out from their hiding places. Gone is their silent vigil. They are harsh calls of warning. Then I hear the howling.

Moments later the wolf has stuck his head right into the tent. My first impression isn't one of danger or fear but of his absolute beauty. He is a great big timber wolf. His tawny head and long front legs with giant-looking furry paws are covered with drops of half-frozen snow that gleam like diamonds on his thick fur. He has a good look around, as though I should have been expecting his visit. Maybe I am. After all, this is his world.

My heart is thundering. Yet my strongest instinct is that he's not going to attack me. I have learned to trust my instinct. It's all I have. I stay quiet, but the wolf knows I'm shaken. You can't pretend to animals. They always know how you feel. Then he backs away and he's gone.

I have to go out to repair the ripped tent flap with duct tape. The moon has risen, revealing a pack of wolves waiting like grey shadows among the trees.

The next morning they have left but they come back again at the end of the day when I set up camp. I am on a desolate road that stretches for miles through the forest. I've only observed one or two vehicles over the last few days travelling to the mines in the far east of Russia. There are no houses for hundreds of miles and I wonder if these wolves have seen a human before. Perhaps I'm just part of the wildlife.

Over the next few days they disappear at daylight and reappear when I stop for the night. They never come close to the tent again or harm me. It is as if they are running with me. They always gather for the night quite a distance away.

I'm uneasy – yet at the same time their presence comforts me in a way I don't quite understand. After about a week they vanish. I believe it's because I've left their terrain; I have crossed an invisible border.

These beautiful wolves with their ancient, strange ways gave me courage to think of the painful memories of why my run had begun.

On 12 June 2002 my husband Clive died in my arms of prostate cancer. I knew with a passionate conviction that I had to do something. To tell people, to remind them to please go for health checks. If Clive and I had thought about him going to the doctor earlier – perhaps he would be with me now. I had to find a way to make others listen, especially men and women who hate going to the doctor and discussing intimate things. There is no social status with cancer. I'm only an ordinary woman, but if I just stayed home doing the weeding in my backyard, nobody would have taken any notice – that's why I am running around the world, and sleeping in the cold in the forests with wolves.

If my message saves even one life – it will all have been worthwhile.

CHAPTER 1

Clive

Tenby, Wales, 2002

We thought he could beat it, just as Clive had always conquered everything. Years ago, he sailed practically everywhere in the world, delivering yachts. He sailed boats no one else could manage. He escaped from pirates on the high seas, weathered all storms. He had always been fit, and very full of life and laughter.

Clive had twinkling blue eyes in an inquisitive and happy face; you could stop to chat to him for a moment – and still be talking hours later. I met him in 1982, when I had been at a low point, struggling to get an old and ramshackle 17ft sailing boat ready to sail solo across the Atlantic. Although he was a businessman in Pembrokeshire, he couldn't stay away from the sea, and was helping out at Kelpie's Boatyard in Pembroke Dock, where he rigged my little boat. Clive had been married before like me and had two deeply loved grown-up children, Jayne and Nigel. I was also very close to Eve and James, my children from my first marriage.

After I completed my solo voyage, we had a simple wedding and nearly twenty extremely happy years together. We would walk or run down to the sea and look at the sunrise, making a golden path of light across the sea from the harbour and North Beach in Tenby where we lived.

'I think heaven isn't later,' he often said. 'Heaven's right here on this earth.'

Half-jokingly, he called doctors 'vets' as a compliment. He loved animals and admired vets who have to look after patients of *all* sizes, including strange animals. I had already run the Sahara Marathon. Clive had made a film about it and about working animals. We had visited a donkey clinic in Marrakesh after the race; my feet were blistered and Clive, worried because no doctor was available, asked their head vet to treat them. The vet had done a terrific job on his first two-legged donkey, applying soothing green cream smelling of aloe vera, normally used for girth galls, he said, while his other patients had eehowed, looking on sympathetically. The blisters healed perfectly.

All these carefree times suddenly ended. Our world changed in a way sadly known by millions but shatteringly new to us. We were unaware of cancer – not of the fearful loss, pain and grief it caused to so many, but that it can happen so easily to anybody. It seems unbelievable now.

On 26 June 2000 Clive went to see Dr Griffiths, his 'vet', at Tenby Surgery, because he had begun to have discomfort when he peed. We were shocked, devastated when the tests showed that Clive had prostate cancer.

'It's not so bad,' Dr Griffiths tried to reassure us. 'It's often one of the easiest cancers to treat. You can have prostate cancer and live to ninety – and then get run over by a bus.'

The next test, the scan, revealed it had already spread into Clive's bones. I prayed for a miracle that night; I would have done anything to have had the cancer instead of him, but Clive just said, 'I can cope with this.'

For the next year, life went on almost as normal. He responded very well to the medication and I couldn't get over his strong will. He began running on the beach, which he had actually never done before – he was not a runner. It was so hard because for a long time he wanted to keep the fact that he was ill between us and his doctors.

One day I saw he wasn't really able to jog on the beach any more but was trying to hide it. Then he stopped and put his arm around me.

'Don't cry,' he said, 'or you'll make me cry too. Be strong.'

He was well enough to go camping in Ireland in the autumn as he had longed to do. It was lovely. The Irish side of my family kept saying how well Clive looked, which made me proud but also tore me apart as I couldn't say what had been happening. Whatever he chose to do *was* the way to do it.

I remember our tent beside the misty dunes, reeds and grasses in the early morning near Rosslare Harbour, before catching the ferry back. We had such fun. Time generously stopped its bitter headlong race; and stood still, just for a little while. It was time's gift that meant everything. Things last for ever, not in years, but in the moments in which they happen.

Clive was as full of dreams and ideas as ever. He eventually told his daughter and son, and a few more people about the cancer, and we carried on as he wanted to do. It wasn't that he didn't want to face his problem; it wasn't about achieving last dreams. Clive and I didn't believe in the word *last*. Dreams are founded on reality and facing up to trouble. We just kept on going forward, because it was the only way.

He wrote a poem, 'I Want to See the World':

> *I want to be a sailor, I want to roam the oceans far and*
>   *wide,*
> *I want to see the islands and the far off distant lands,*
> *To listen to the music of the drum.*
> *I want to ride on camels, and elephants too,*
> *And lie on beaches basking in the sun.*
> *I want to go to India, and see the famous Tajah,*
> *Then visit Everest and its peaks …*

Much later, on my world run, I realised that it was Clive who taught me that you never give yourself a break going uphill but only when you are over the top of the mountain. And that the mountains are in the mind.

Clive longed to go to Nepal. He had been born in India and his father had been in the British Army in charge of the Gurkhas. Clive had never gone back because he hadn't wanted to go as a tourist. Before his illness he had accepted an invitation by the Nepal Trust for us to trek and help them build a hospital in Humla. He still said he'd do anything to go. He also wanted to go to Cuba to make a film about a run, as he had done in the Sahara.

He very nearly made it to Cuba too. He felt better and insisted I go ahead and come back and fetch him after the run, so he could just film it in a few days. He reckoned he'd be OK for a few days away.

This was never going to happen.

Suddenly he got much worse. In January 2002, we were lying in bed together. I had been dozing and Clive pulled the duvet – that's all he did – and his arm gave a loud crack.

'I think it's broken,' he said. 'It's OK if I just lie still.'

The ambulance came. At the hospital they said that the break above the elbow was a classic sign of bone cancer spreading out of control. He was in and out of hospital until April, bravely going to physiotherapy to get back what strength he could. Doing exercises as prescribed by the doctor, with his arm in a sling. I saw it all. I went everywhere with him.

The physiotherapists were astonished he could joke. He used to say, 'Oh, I have *everything* going for me. My teeth are going, my hair's going, my eyes are going …'

On 10 April, his birthday, he ate his cake, or a bit of it. I gave him a little torch you could hold in the palm of your hand. He gave it back, saying, 'Please keep this for me.'

From soon after his birthday he was in hospital until towards the very end.

Peter Hutchinson of PHD Designs, who make the finest lightweight down clothing on earth, sent Clive a down vest weighing only 250 grams which sat on his fragile bones, giving him so much comfort.

After the arm, his hip broke. Just as they were hoping to get him walking again, the tumours in his spine caused his legs to become paralysed.

He bore it all, as everyone does, and still tried to have a laugh. When his friend Chester visited, asking if there was anything Clive needed, he replied, 'Yes, I need a fast car.'

Ward 10 Palliative and Cancer Care Ward, in our local Withybush Hospital in Haverfordwest, is a place I will never forget, of endless empathy and caring, of a lightness and kindness beyond words. Anne Barnes, a gifted and blessed cancer specialist, always wore not medical gear but bright clothes to cheer her patients up. When Clive and others were transferred to her ward she often dropped dark hints about the latest sexual orgies and parties in Ward 10 at 2am. Of course these didn't ever happen but the thought brought a smile to her patients' faces and may have hidden their terrible pain better than the morphine.

The most dedicated nurses I have ever known let me sleep in my sleeping bag for long months, or even on the edge of Clive's bed, just holding him. One night I awoke and found Clive looking at me. He smiled and said, 'You had such a good sleep.' There was a look of pride and love in his eyes I can't express. The nurses patiently taught me how to do everything for Clive such as cleaning and washing him. It was a privilege for me to do it: I would have done anything for him.

Their policy was to enable patients to come home for the final days if the patient wished for it. I shall never forget how caringly they went about it. They even had a special hospital bed brought to our home, and round-the-clock nursing care.

Clive was so happy to see the honeysuckle he had planted and smiled at the sight of the sparrows, which he always called his 'feathered hooligans', feasting on fat balls outside the bedroom window. I had actually been training them up with extra food before he came home so they could put on a gala show. A day later, 12 June 2002, he was gone.

After all the pain and suffering, I awoke beside him feeling that a light had come on. He had been given all his strength and spirit back and was moving on.

When the kind lady doctor had been and the wonderful young Paul Sartori nurse (like our local Macmillan's nurses) had retired next door after hugging me, I just held Clive close to me all through the night. I didn't know what else to do. I held him like you might hold onto someone in a desert.

He was off on such a long journey; he might be lonely for a little while. I was on a journey too. Beginning a journey and ending a journey. I was heartbroken, and held him and looked at him all those hours; and then I knew you can only keep hold of beauty by letting it go.

He *had* won his battle right to the very end. You don't win a battle because of how it turns out. You win by the way you face it. He was up among the pirates. He was happy.

Even during this desperate fight Clive had never lost his sense of fun. My monument to him shouldn't be sorrowful, grieving or gloomy. I had to do something for Clive that would be crazy and huge. I could run some marathons for cancer awareness, I thought.

I had been looking at the map of the world on my wall, wondering if I could afford overseas marathons, when something took hold of me by the scuff of the neck; a thought broke through my grief and seized every part of my being.

I would run around the world instead.

CHAPTER 2

The Plan

Tenby, August 2002

I was born in Davos, Switzerland, where my mother was in a clinic suffering from tuberculosis, while my father was away serving in the British Army. When I was two days old the doctors put an advertisement in the local paper for a foster mother, as my mother couldn't look after me. There were 45 applicants as I learned many years later. My mother chose the local postman's wife, who was good to me. To strengthen my lungs, my foster mother took me for long walks, which ended up in the grounds of the TB clinic so my mother could look at me out of her window, because her infection made it impossible for her to have physical contact with me. I have shadowy memories of the faces of my mother and foster mother and the black squirrels eating nuts off my hands. My foster mother always dressed me beautifully and had photos of me taken for my poor mother to have around her bedside later.

I never knew my mother, but I shall always feel such huge love and gratitude to her for having the courage to give birth to me when she was so ill, and also for her greater courage in having to face giving me away. I feel I owe my life to many exceptional, caring and loving people.

When I was two my mother sadly died and my Anglo-Irish grandmother, who was called Carlie, came to collect me to live with her in Country Limerick, Ireland. She gave me a rabbit called Peter, and took me away. She broke the link. My last memory of my foster mother was of a lady with hair in a brown bun crying as she ran beside the train taking me away. From then on Carlie cared for me even though she became crippled with osteoarthritis.

In 1951 when I was five my father, a tall charismatic army officer with kind eyes, married a marvellous Swiss French lady – Marianne. Carlie was bedridden by this time, but my father felt that I was happy with her and it would be unsettling to move me, so we kind of looked after each other. In those long ago days in Ireland, life was simply worked out in the way that everybody thought best. I don't regret it. In 1957 my father also died, leaving Marianne to raise their four children. He was only 47.

Although I never moved in with them, Marianne, whose riverside cottage was a few yards down the road from Grandmother Carlie, kept a loving eye on me. Marianne had a very tough struggle to bring up her four children alone. She was proud and very hardworking. She gave French lessons, sewing lessons, dancing lessons, anything to make ends meet. We became very close after I grew up.

The strange thing is that although Marianne is not really my mother and did not bring me up, we are very alike in character. Marianne is the head of the family today and is the foundation of the happiness of my own children and grandchildren. I love and admire Marianne and her children unconditionally – my half-sister Maude and half-brothers Gerald, Nicolas and Ronnie.

Carlie needed me and I was the only person to whom she really responded and was kind. Crippled and bedridden with osteoarthritis, she would thump the floor at night with her stick for me to come to her aid. I would feel so helpless, listening to her screaming for hours with the terrible pain that pills couldn't ease. I loved her but remember my anger and sorrow as I tried to push her across the gap between her commode and the bed, praying she wouldn't fall. Although just a child, I was already her carer. Her nurses seldom stayed as she was difficult with everybody except me.

Carlie guided me in many ways. She was very religious and for years tutored me herself. I didn't go to school regularly until I was thirteen. But above all she taught me that freedom and responsibility go together, that life is the best university and that anyone can reach for anything.

'Rosie,' she would say, 'it's not good looks or natural gifts that count – luckily for you my girl! – it's the wanting to do things that makes them happen.'

I was tall, thin and gangling with long pigtails.

To do my English essay, she'd send me off on my donkey Jeanette, and then I would have to write about my adventures to entertain her. It was Carlie's influence that set me off on a lifetime of adventures.

Carlie had been a keen gardener in her youth and she still tried somehow to carry on gardening – through me, so to speak – from her bedroom. Slugs and snails brought in, along with all the greenery, would tumble onto her floor. Furiously, with knotted crippled fingers, she'd help me bunch flowers. It had to be done just so. The trumpets of the daffodils all had to point one way. Sometimes the room would be wall-to-wall with daffodils, forget-me-nots or even buttercups and dandelions. She sent me to Limerick with her long-suffering lowly paid gardener to sell them to eke out our funds. It was great for her – one of the few physical ways she could be a bit independent and earn money from bed. We were far from wealthy as there was no National Health Service in Ireland, and her medicines were very expensive.

When I used to go to Limerick market to sell the flowers for her, I would also take bunches of flowers from my own little flower bed to sell, as my dream was to save up to buy a pony. I secretly sold most of my clothes at a secondhand shop too, but I never really managed to save more than a pound or two for the horse. Animals were my life and love.

Nobody talked about the past. Maybe Marianne, so sweet-natured, could have done so, but I couldn't stand the aura of pain, nor the sympathy. My grandmother would never talk about how she'd found me or about my past. It took me years to learn about it all. It caused her too much pain. She hated looking back, but even though her own prospects were so bleak she did look forward with all her might to the future, which she said was through me. Her strong ideas will always be what I most remember about her.

I had been brought up with animals because Carlie was certain that it is animals that give you respect for life. Mostly we collected orphans. I ended up with the elderly Jeanette and four little motherless donkey foals, bought for about five shillings from farmers who did not want to keep them; a little dog called Bobby; seven goats; a chicken with one leg; and a beautiful dairy cow called Cleopatra, who gave good milk even though she was elderly. As I did not have a horse I taught Cleopatra to wear a saddle and halter – and rode her on one occasion, to the Pony Club. Of course we came last because cows jump over the moon only in fairy stories – but we did have a rosette tied to her tail, after trying hard in the gymkhana, even though I fell off at the end as cows trot and gallop with their heads down. With Cleopatra as my steed, falling off was especially uncomfortable as she had a pair of very pretty but quite sharp horns! Anyway, animals were my education – and I could not have had a better one.

I did get a horse in the end, in a way I could never have dreamed. When I was aged about nine, all the local children were asked to the country estate of a rather grand lady called Mrs De Vere for a picnic and summer fete. We were given rides on an old black mare who was led up and down by the gardener. The mare was very unhappy about this, and kept trying to snap and bite everyone, even biting the gardener's trousers as he gave a leg up, but I just fell in love with her. She was tall – about 16 hands high – and very fat, fierce and wild looking. I remember going to an old oak tree with all the other children and being told we could have a wish here as it was a lucky tree. I wished with all my heart that Columbine, as she was called, could be mine.

Amazingly, three months later, the old mare arrived right at my front door with her saddle and bridle, led by the gardener. He explained that Mrs de Vere wouldn't let him ride her any more as he was too heavy and because the mare was very old – and that is why the lady had decided to give Columbine to me. She thought I had a special way with animals, as I was the only child Columbine had not tried to bite!

The mare was so big that she more or less took charge of me and brought me up – she was my friend for years. It was fun teaching my sister Maude, just four years younger than me, how to ride on her.

When I was young I dreamed of being a runner, but thought I was no good. I'd never believed I could run a marathon, still less run around the world. Then, when I was about 47, I picked up a copy of *Runner's World* in a doctor's surgery while awaiting an inoculation. Having read the torn copy of the magazine, I thought, *I can do that*, and that very evening set off to run around the block.

A year later in 1995 I decided to enter the London Marathon and started to train for it. One day I was struggling hard up a steep hill thinking I was crazy to attempt a marathon when two super-fit local runners caught up with me and said, 'Hey, you're doing pretty well.' They slowed down to stay with me and we ran together the rest of the way. They taught me to believe in myself just as Carlie used to do, and that made all the difference.

After the London Marathon I became aware of the Swiss Alpine Marathon in Davos. I thought it would be a wonderful opportunity to go back to my birthplace. When I mentioned to the race organisers that I'd spent my early childhood in Davos they ran an article looking for my foster mother. I had had never been in touch with her as my grandmother had not wished to talk about the past, and had never told me her full name. They found her – Frieda Fridli who now, at 98, was the oldest person in Davos. That didn't prevent her from coming to the finish. She invited me to her home – and she had photos of me as a baby on her mantelpiece. It was as if she had waited specially to see me again. I was so proud to introduce her to Clive, who had come with me as photographer, and we stayed in touch with her until she died at the age of 100.

It made me realize that running is far more than a sport, it is a way of communication. Running had brought me back to my past all those years ago and suddenly I was sure it would help me move forward and honour Clive's final battle too.

I spent hours looking at maps. I saw that I could run *all* the way round the world without having to cross any oceans. It would have to be through icy northern latitudes, the harshest latitudes on earth, but it took hold of my mind and spun it in circles of excitement. It also looked cheaper than other ways because … it *was* cheaper than other ways. It was the package tour alone on foot. No expensive long-haul airfares.

I threw myself into planning it. The preparations were to take more than a year. With hindsight, I should perhaps have spent longer, but it just seemed very important that I should go as soon as possible: I'd had Clive on my mind, and also all those faces in Ward 10; people who had dreams, people who had led careful lives and had made plans for the future, which they now could not achieve.

I thought I could run from my own front door to London and Harwich, take the ferry to the Hook of Holland, then across Europe to Moscow all the way through Siberia. The next sea after the English Channel on this route would be the short stretch across the Bering Sea. Then I'd reach the immense wilderness of the far north of Alaska, head across the North American continent to Nova Scotia then Greenland and across the north of Iceland, and finally down the length of Great Britain back to my front door. It was like a voyage on two feet. I *had* to go for it.

It broke my heart to think how for years fate had, without my knowing it, been training me up for this but hadn't warned me in time about the cancer. Yet these earlier expeditions, like sailing the Atlantic single handed, had given me strength and knowledge. I feel blessed to have been alone on the ocean trying to look beyond the horizon and to navigate by the stars. The voyage had taken 70 days because the boat had been so small and old. During this time I had not seen a human face nor a tree nor any land; I hoped that had taught me to deal with loneliness I would feel on this journey too. Hard lessons from the past can be valuable. Also, between taking up running in 1995 and Clive's death in 2002, I had run marathons but had often used running as a way of travelling and researching countries for my writing. The journeys were short – around six weeks each and about 1000 miles per journey – in countries that included Albania, Romania, Iceland and war-torn Kosovo.

Because these were self-financed or with just a small commission from *Runner's World*, I had to be self-sufficient, carry a backpack and live in a tent – and do all this on a small budget. I had learnt to curl up and sleep like an animal by the side of the road – and hoped to do the same on this expedition. The world run was just going to be a longer version of my earlier ones.

My local running club, TROT St Clears (TROT stands for Taf Running and Orienteering Team), encouraged and helped me so much. I began training by running in races in the Welsh hills. I'd bring the bivvi and camp the night before. I found comfort in sleeping under the stars and began to understand: I didn't need to fight my grief, and I didn't have to be ashamed of sorrow – it isn't a weakness. All these things became clearer when I was outside in the wide open spaces, amid the beauty of stars and moon and dawn, and even in the rain. The tall grass seemed to touch the moon. Once I had stopped in the dark, after arriving late by bus, and was a bit too near a footpath, and someone walking his dog in the early morning nearly trod on me. It gave us both a fright.

Next I ran the Cardiff Marathon in August 2002. About halfway through the marathon I tripped into a pothole and fell bang wallop on the tarmac – definitely *not* much of a prospect for running in the wilds at this time! Yet although blood began dripping down onto the road as I had cut my face, I was suddenly aware that my legs felt fine. I could run faster and it didn't hurt.

I think I may have helped some of the other competitors to keep going when they were exhausted. Maybe they thought, *She's going on even though she's bleeding!* I hope I didn't kill someone that way, but I made it to the finish. It was amazing. My name was called and I got first prize in the over-50 category. I had a black eye and swollen cheek and when the local newspaper photographer came to take a picture, I asked him, 'Do you want my best profile?' as I held ice to my face and tried to eat a banana at the same time.

We looked at each other and started laughing. That was when I realised that I hadn't laughed properly for months. I knew Clive would have wanted it. He spent his last year putting things in place so that I could move forward. He was a private person and he wanted me to raise cancer awareness, but it was as important to him as my doing the run that it should not be a morbid journey; he would be proud to have inspired my run as he did, but he would hate it to be all about him or sentimental. Our feelings were and are very personal. So my run would be looking forward – running not from but towards life, as he would have wished.

Even though we did not discuss my run, he knew I would do something. He had repeatedly told me he wanted me to live with courage. I would not die inside and I would not dishonour Clive by treating my journey as a 20,000 mile round-the-world funeral procession. I would grab life double for him, feel love more, be more. If someone you love grabs life for you and flies the banner for you, death can be defeated.

All this gave me strength through that first summer. I knew that what I wanted to do was going to happen.

'You'll succeed, Mum,' said my daughter Eve, 'because you have people who care deeply about you.'

My revered stepmother Marianne was on the phone the moment she heard I was going to do the world run. 'I'll be waiting for you in Tenby at the finish,' she said. Marianne is now in her early eighties. She still lives in Ireland, drives a car like a racing driver and teaches French in County Limerick to university level.

My son James had already started thinking about the rosiearoundtheworld website. The plan was that charities would be linked to the website and people could send money in; also if I was given money I would pass it on, but I would not ask for it, as I would have my work cut out just surviving, and also I would be in the wilderness and in some of the poorest countries in the world. Even so, I hoped I would be in a unique position to help with cancer awareness by doing my run around the world.

I didn't have much money but I did have fabulous sponsors of equipment that I had used for years and the backing and friendship of *Runner's World*. I didn't attempt to try and secure large financial sponsorship, as I felt I would not succeed and that I might spend all my savings just trying to get it. Above all, I was still much too sad to ask anyone I did not already know. The thought of discussing Clive's death and details for sponsorship with strangers was something that appalled me, and I would not do it.

But I did have a fabulous 'A-Team'. Eve, James and my great friend Catherine in London got going with the research. Catherine also got her beloved cat Nedd to cross his lucky black paws for me.

Steven Seaton, publisher of *Runner's World UK*, had always encouraged me to write by commissioning pieces about my running adventures in the past, such as my run across Romania when I'd met all the vampires. I didn't even have to ask before he said that *Runner's World* would sponsor me.

Ann Rowell, one of my best running friends, offered to do my accounts and keep an eye on things while I was gone as my family lived far away. She would also fend off the bailiffs by paying bills from my account. She and another great friend with whom I used to go running, Kath Garner, had joint Power of Attorney, drawn up by my solicitor. Ann optimistically said this was useful because they could go and rescue me if 'I became unconscious and senseless in Siberia'.

Ann also suggested that Matt Evans, an amazing runner who ran ten marathons in ten days, manage the rental of my house through his company, the Pembrokeshire Coastal Cottages Holiday Letting Business. It was sound advice. I would need all the income I could get.

As for equipment, I asked those whose kit I had used and trusted for years for their advice, and they helped me without question. Saucony UK sponsored my shoes; Peter Hutchinson and his team at PHD Designs in Staybridge designed the sleeping-bag system that allowed a temperature-range of 100° on the run, from the little down Minimus bag for the summer weighing only 450gm to the extreme cold-weather sleeping bags that would save my life at temperatures colder than −60°C.

Terra Nova, whose products I've also used for years, sponsored the tents for the journey, including their invaluable Saturn bivvi, my home for the whole of the first winter, weighing only 2lb 2oz. I had a thirst-point filter bottle so I could drink any water; and so on. Such simple things would make a huge difference.

I had to really plan what I was going to take. Even small, down-to-earth items were important, such as face care. All I took was sun block and Vaseline – later to be replaced by whatever its local equivalent was in any country I happened to be in – and my wonderful friend Eva Fraser, who runs the Facial Fitness Clinic in London, taught me facial exercises to help circulation, looks, mental attitude and how to care for my face without carrying jars and potions. Every part of the body is important.

Getting my Russian visa was a problem. Because of the length of my run the only type of visa that would work was a one-year Russian 'business' visa, but as the manager of one of the agencies pointed out, there aren't many business meetings in the depths of the Siberian forests and the people who arranged things for him in Russia would get into trouble. The police would have them and me up without question. I'd be put in jail. The letters of commission and good character, provided by *Runner's World*, my book agents Watson, Little Ltd and the organisers of the Daily Telegraph Adventure Show I'd proudly presented, seemed to frighten the agencies even more because they made it clear that I was serious about the run. Someone suggested I just say I was 'going to Russia to do research' on running, but I decided I had to be straightforward as to why I wanted the visa: it was the only way to manage anything regarding visas and papers, and it was vitally important that it was all properly arranged.

As part of my training, I ran another marathon – the Loch Ness Marathon – in September 2002. I was getting fitter and used to being outdoors all the time. I could feel at home anywhere. The night before the race I camped the night beside Loch Ness. The water sparkled as the stars came out, looking mysterious enough for one to believe anything. I thought of putting biscuits out for Nessie but fell asleep instead so she never came to visit after all.

I was lucky enough to get booked to give a few talks to help with funds and to begin promoting cancer awareness.

An especially memorable occasion was a lunch function at the Bolton and Bury Chamber of Commerce. I was training hard now, and had gone running and camping in the hills the night before, getting my one good blouse all crumpled as I had lain on it by mistake. No problem. I ran down into Bury town early and popped into McDonald's because they have nice hard seats in the cafe where I could sit on the blouse to iron it. I was very pleased with the 'ironing' and got a bit carried away and decided to wash my hair in the 'Ladies' while I was at it. Unfortunately I got my head stuck in the machine on the wall on which there were signs saying 'soap … hot air … water'. To my relief, two girls came in and rescued me, so that was fine. The hazards of modern life! But it taught me a valuable lesson in the gentle 'art of making do' or improvisation that was going to be very useful during my run.

The talks helped boost my courage. The Chairman of the Chamber even posed with the Saucony shoes around his neck along with his golden chain to show solidarity with my goals, and then they put them around my neck for a photo for their journal and stood there cheering me – while a bishop who was there blessed the shoes, wishing for God to go with me – as indeed he did.

By now I was beyond feeling excited or apprehensive; I had no time to be introspective. Every single second was taken up getting ready to go, thinking about it, trying to get everything right.

At Christmas I stayed at home, spending hours calling my family, then set off on my fine new bicycle, bought for me by my friends Chester and Jean in Pembroke Dock. I passed much of the day cycling, visiting friends, only spending a little time with them, and then on to the next – being careful not to drink too much wine! I couldn't quite yet bear sharing a whole family Christmas – it hurt somehow – but then suddenly in the New Year I knew that Clive was happy, having a riot of fun up in heaven, and that I didn't have to worry. He was with his friends.

I decided to set off in October 2003. I'd have to run through the European winter to Moscow but that would give me the whole of the first summer to get through as much of treacherous Siberia as I could before winter came again.

Siberia derives its name from 'Siber' – land without end – and that is what it's like. I could not escape the Siberian winter since it is so vast and the distances too great, but I wanted to run across as much of it as possible before the extreme cold set in. It was likely to be –40 or –50°C but the temperatures could plummet as low as –70°C in Eastern Siberia.

I planned my route, through Holland, Germany, Poland, Lithuania, Latvia to Riga, and then from Riga to Moscow and on from there to Siberia – and beyond. I did not have the big Russian visa yet, but was working on it. For Lithuania and Latvia, British subjects do not require visas. If the Russian visa problem got solved, there was just a slight possibility that I might run from Poland through Russian Kallingrad to get to Riga, as it was shorter than going through Lithuania and Latvia, but time would tell.

My house-plants grew to the ceiling, thriving on neglect. The house dusted itself. I made a pot of stew once a week, eating it all the time, and got out so many maps and plans the living-room floor was always covered with them so you couldn't see any carpet to Hoover anyway.

The planning and preparation for my world run were all-consuming and there were promises to keep before I even set off. Clive and I had planned to trek in Nepal in aid of the Nepal Trust and the Rotary's Club's work in the isolated Himalayas. When he had been very sick, he had asked me to go up to the big Rotary Conference in Glasgow – and I promised the audience of 2000 that we would go to Nepal when he was better. As he had not been able to do so – I had to do this myself.

So in April just for six weeks, I left on this strange tangent. It was high-altitude training that was valuable, but it was much more than that. Liz and Jim Donovan, who run the Nepal Trust, invited me to run and trek to fulfil Clive's dearest wish. Maybe Clive's persistent desire that he might make it, even when very ill, was a kind of foreknowledge that it would help me, as well as helping the extraordinary work of the Nepal Trust. The small charity, together with huge input by Rotary International, have brought health, literacy and income to people in the forgotten high Himalayas at Humla and other especially remote places, targeting areas where need is greatest. They had steadfastly continued this even during the civil war in Nepal that killed 10,000 people in the previous eight years.

Accompanied by 20 young Nepalese men and women, tough and fast as Gurkhas, I 'speed-trekked' over 32 mountain passes to Everest Base Camp. Even though we kept getting held up by Maoists, we did 1750km in 68 days, raising the money for the hospital and clinics.

Through the Nepal Trust I met Liza Hollinghead, who runs the Ecologia Travel Company, founded to help fund the Kitezh Community for Children in Russia, which looks after orphans rescued from heartbreaking situations. I was so inspired to be helping both these charities that I added them to the causes, along with cancer awareness, that I was going to support on my run. Dedicated and determined, Liza managed to get me the long-term Russian visa where everybody else had failed.

My worries about having no contacts in Siberia were also sorted when I spotted an ad in a running magazine for the Siberian Marathon taking place on 3 August. *Woman's Weekly* commissioned me to write an article, so I'd have enough money to go for the marathon. In Omsk I stayed with Elena in her neat home in a crumbling apartment, learning quite a lot about life in Western Siberia during my few days there.

Omsk is a beautiful city, but life is hard here. People clean their water by filtering and repeatedly straining and boiling it for three days before it's safe to drink or make a cup of tea.

They are too poor to replace the old Soviet factories upriver which empty dangerous chemicals into the water. It looks clean to the eye but is often toxic and there's a high incidence of cancer here, I was told. Doctors fight this battle even though the wages of a doctor are so low that a doctor has to have several jobs to survive – and the hospital has few facilities. I was so glad to be running the Siberian Marathon in aid of the Siberian Railway Hospital after I visited it. The head doctor blithely described how he'd cut a patient open, put his guts onto a sterilised plate, removed the rotten bits and popped them back before sewing him up. The patient recovered fine.

People really put everything out for the Siberian Marathon. Bright stalls selling all kinds of things were set up and flags flown. Everyone lined the streets, cheering so loudly from the first mile, just as in the London Marathon.

I'd have to run 6000 miles before I next saw Omsk, but I had a home and good friends there already. I was also very lucky to meet Geoff Hall, the only other British runner, who even allowed me to take his photo for *Woman's Weekly*. Geoff became an exceptional supporter of my run, coordinating my equipment from the UK, sending me shoes and other kit to isolated parts of the world, and making all the difference. It was amazing that I went all the way to Siberia to meet one of the British lynchpins of my whole run.

After the race, as the plane took off, with the crimson of an exquisite Siberian sunrise bathing the circle of the horizon, my heart was full and I had so much to think about. I knew I had to find out more; and that between Nepal and

Kitezh and the Siberian Railway Hospital, the world is vast
– so very, very vast.

Finally, on 2 October 2003 after all the dreaming and schem-
ing and planning and preparation, the day arrived. I stood in
front of my house in Tenby, among friends, ready to set off.
I had decided to leave on that date because it was my birthday, my 57th to be precise.

There wasn't much fuss – round-the-world sailor Sir
Francis Chichester used to say: 'The celebrations come *after*
the voyage' – but my son James was there, my brother Nicolas who had come over specially from Ireland, some close
local friends, running pals and a few others, such as Chas
and Carol, the owners of Tenby Autoparts. Chas had shared
many a joke and tall story with Clive while he'd been getting
bits and pieces for Cassidy, our elderly campervan.

My brother Nicolas drew the outline of my foot on the
flagstone in the gateway to my house – *the first step*. The plan
was that the *last* step of my run would be in Tenby on the
same flagstone after I circled the world.

Everything happened so fast. The local telly filmed me,
everyone kissed me and off I set. I ran down the street,
around the next corner and then I was gone.

CHAPTER 3

The Tenby Bear

Wales, 2 October 2003

It's only after I've run two miles that I remember it's my birthday. I never ate the cake I found hidden at the back of the fridge last night, or waited for the champagne.

It's so strange to be running up the hill to New Hedges and Pentlepoir, seeing the sublime and beautiful sea, and cliffs and coastal path my friends and I have run along so many times in stormy weather, on rainy days and in magical days of sunshine like this morning. Surely I'm running just a short run along these familiar ways and will be back home in time for breakfast. I'm looking at everything around me with passion and intensity, knowing it's for the last time for maybe years. Everything seems different looking at it for the last time: the colours brighter in the beautiful gardens of the cottages and in the green, green fields: the scurries of the first golden leaves on the roadside being chased by the breeze; the smell of sun on grass.

I think back to my house, where my son James and brother Nicolas are getting ready to go as they have to leave soon to return to their homes. The momentum has swept us on. I want to say goodbye again. Yet this is partly the purpose of this run; to go forwards and not back on an easy track when you feel lonely; just as it's always been for people on slow journeys and voyages long ago.

A shy little girl rushes out from her home with her mother to give me a painting she's done for me and some sweets. A bouncy lady with twinkling eyes and Indian summer sunburn on her cheeks makes fresh sandwiches for me.

'Oh I'm so proud of you,' she says. 'Keep going. You're insane, you need to see the doctor, but don't go before you've done the run, you don't want to see the light too soon.'

The feelings of day one are encapsulated by the enormity of what lies ahead. Captured in the essence of burning feet, pain and flashes of joy and happiness, and lovely people. As Darwin wrote in one of his journals, 'To be a traveller is to see the goodness everywhere.'

I manage 25 miles to just beyond Carmarthen the first day, but often have to sit down by the side of the road to rub my feet, burning from the pressure of running on tarmac with the very heavy pack. I need a fire extinguisher.

My head is swimming with emotion at what I've left behind, and excitement at what lies ahead. It sets a precedent that I am too exhausted to go into the town and look up people who have kindly asked me to stay. So I put up the bivvi among tall grass and bushes in the centre of a piece of wasteland and I go to sleep at once. I wake up in the middle of the night with my head sticking out of the bivvi, looking up at the stars and wondering where on earth I am. Then I realise – I am on my way. I feel overwhelmed with both joy and sadness …

I pray that I can achieve what I need to do. I don't feel strong, but very determined, with a mixture of physical and mental determination, like at the start of my transatlantic voyage that has now become my 'Voyage on Two Feet'. The tide is running with me and there's no going back. The first step, I've done the first step, and that's the longest step of all.

I can't go back; I must avoid injury. All this makes the first few miles feel nerve-racking, heart-stopping. I think about the vastness of what lies ahead and tell myself, *You only have to run for an hour … and then another hour after that … Do not think of it as a great big deal all at once …* I think of it in steps … I can do one step … And then the next one … And the next one …

As always on adventures – at sea or on land on two feet – this journey is a mixture of dreams: something that sends a shiver down my spine, that I have to do and, practical realities. It's nothing airy-fairy, but facts that make dreams come true. I've already become trained at staying out at night over the past months; the difference now is that I am really on my way. I have to look after myself, and will have to do so for a long, long time.

Big chunks of lead seem to have got into my backpack. Forget all the training runs I've been on with 5kg or 10kg packs of potatoes to teach me to run with weight. Forget sessions laden with my kit; you never quite take *all* the kit when you know you're going home to a nice warm bed. I'm carrying stuff for the winter that I've been afraid to send ahead of me in case I lose it – and on top of this, I have a bear.

He's the Tenby Bear, come along to protect me. He even wears a little green knitted jacket with *'Tenby's Bear'* written on it. The children at one of our local schools want him to look after me and he's my talisman. Next day, as I run to Cross Hands, I feel better, having managed to post back a little of my kit that I don't need so much. But Tenby Bear stays. He's not heavy, he's my brother.

There are seven days in Wales: exquisite hills, wild sea in Carmarthen Bay, glorious autumn colours in the woodlands of Wentworth. I run through Cross Hands and am invited by some pleasant-looking ladies to attend a murder. I wonder what dastardly skulduggery is being planned but it's just a village-hall play called *The Murder*.

Running with a heavy pack is better than a lullaby. I have a lovely day with friends in Newport, meeting up with Mike Rowland, a marathon coach and one of the best artists in Wales. I'm so tired I go to sleep in another classroom while he's teaching. I don't even wake up when they test the fire-alarm. He finds me curled up fast asleep, about to get locked in for the night by mistake.

On 8 October, I run across the Severn Bridge after picking up some Welsh Oak leaves to keep forever with me.

That's it. I've done Wales. Now for the rest of the world.

CHAPTER 4

Eyes in Your Feet

England–Holland–Germany, October 2003

Choppy waves in the fresh breeze. Darkness falls as I gaze back at England.

It's 225 miles since I crossed the Severn Bridge. Seagulls cry as the ferry pulls out. I'm standing on deck, looking as the lights come on in Harwich, and darkness falls.

'October blackberries are the Devil's fruit,' my grandmother Carlie used to say but I think they're the most tempting of any fruit. They make handy fuelling stations for a runner and I feast on them. There has been a full moon above the sweeping soft English autumn countryside and the days are sparkling and sunny though sometimes chilly. It's been a beautiful run.

Among the most powerful images of this part of the route are the distinguished buildings and grounds of great stately-looking places like the Marlborough Public School buildings and grounds, and quaint houses and tiny cottages in quiet villages and small market towns like Castle Combe, Chipping Sodbury and others. Even Slough, which I have always only driven through, I now see in a new way too.

Everywhere I'm cheered on and helped with good humour and kindness; especially outside pubs along the canal path from Slough to London, where people sit with their pints, their reflections in the clear water turning them into double pints. En route, I see foxes and badgers, and the blackbird's morning song follows me everywhere.

I have the same feelings that I did when leaving Wales: England, the whole of the British Isles, is so precious and beautiful. My ears ache with listening and trying to remember the melody of the blackbirds and my eyes and mind hurt with storing the sights around me that I will not see again for years.

Near Marlborough in Wiltshire, a vet stops his car. His name is Martin and he tells me he's also a runner. When he ran from Land's End to John O'Groats he used a baby-jogger.

'Much easier than carrying a backpack. You're carrying too much weight which long term will ruin your back. You need to get a cart to pull.'

Looking back, I really respected his advice and wished I'd taken it sooner. At the time, though, I thought it could be difficult to camp at night and progress through tracks in woods with a cart.

It means so much that Mark, Clive's favourite nephew, his wife Mandy and son Andrew drive out to see me. They are such a part of it all, and yet so already is Geoff who I have only ever met once before, at the Omsk Marathon. Geoff runs 20 miles with me and we drink cool lemonade at the end. The most special moments are the two nights with Eve,

Pete and my grandson Michael, after I've run the canal path from Slough to London. I wake up in the spare bedroom, thinking *I have all the time in the world.*

Please make time stand still – also please make time pass that I can win through. There's no point in feeling selfish about this. So many people go through the same thing when they are off on some mission – or off to war. This run is a joy for me to do, but it is also my small personal and fierce war, my little contribution to life, not much compared to what many do. If I was a doctor or nurse I would not run around the world because then I could do more here.

I love my family so much. Eve is like me but much cleverer and more beautiful; Michael is a kindred spirit, though only one and half; Pete's a Liverpudlian, a designer – one of the best people I've ever met. They want me to go on my run; it's for Clive, but it is for them too.

I also feel very sad when saying goodbye to Catherine in London, and to dear Nedd, the black cat who owns her; I have faith I will see them all again; I have faith it will all work out; but my heart is thudding with the immensity of the journey ahead.

I spend several days running from London to Colchester and on to the east coast. I keep thinking, 'This is just one little step, one little breath, in my aim to circle the globe. I have planned it, prepared for it; been inspired to do it; yet it is still something I never thought I could reach for in my lifetime. It has been full of practical, prosaic plans and strategies and solutions; but still something beyond all the horizons I know.

*   *   *

By 19 October, I'm boarding the ferry to Holland.

The ferry docks at Hook at 4am in the stillness of pre-dawn darkness. I unwrap the bivvi, rest in it awhile, awaken to skies blazing in a tangerine sunrise. The huge clouds across the skies are golden. I understand why in Holland they call clouds 'the Dutch mountains'. They are the most spectacular peaks around. Soon, early light is reflecting the tops of many glasshouses in town, which sparkle like diamonds. Thousands appear on bikes on their way to work. Everybody is warm and good-humoured, saying good morning to me in English. There's the smell of hot coffee, fresh croissants and cakes in the chocolatiers and bakeries.

I begin the 50km run to Haarlem. The path is through a forest, then along dykes and canals. A mist descends. Boats emerging out of the fog seem close enough to touch. It almost seems I'm travelling beside them in the same element, on the water. There are misty windmills, endless dykes. I've been to Holland several times, but it's never felt like this. I realise, through the two-week run in Holland, it's the way of travelling that matters. I bless the heavy pack that's crippling me, because I'm so slow. Slowness gives you eyes in your feet and can be a catalyst for the senses.

Klaas Hoeve is publishing two of my sailing books in Dutch. He and his assistant Madelon take me to lunch in Haarlem, bringing chocolate whose giant chocolate letters say *Rosie*. He's meeting me again in the north of Holland at Leewarden. I eat one letter of my name every day for extra energy, continuing along little roads and paths weaving through marshlands, dykes and more empty landscape than I imagined existed in Holland in a misty landscape of sudden shafts of light, with rainstorms, windmills and farms often only just visible as if on a delicate, washed-out artist's canvas.

I'm using a lot of energy and need to eat often. I buy food in little shops in isolated villages. Grocers are understanding when I purchase just a few potatoes, three carrots, one onion. Vegetables are delicious but heavy to carry. It changes my way of shopping completely when I have to carry it all on my back. I'm also rediscovering spaghetti – wonderful with Dutch cheese. There are 500gm per pack and 100gm is 300 calories. If you add various bits and pieces, it's a good budget meal. My tiny stove becomes the centre of my life. There aren't many cafes in the countryside, even in Holland. Even if I find a restaurant, I often don't stop. I must economise as my budget for the entire run is very small. A few thousand pounds a year.

The first frost comes on 23 October: a scattering of snow followed by driving sleet and rain. I'm happy I've picked up a parcel of heavier-duty clothes and kit sent ahead to my publisher. The weather is always good from inside a PHD Khumbu storm-proof Gortex jacket.

On 25 October I run across the first 15km of the Afsluit-dijk dam that stretches 35km in a beautiful, dramatic way between the open water of Waddensee and the inland Ijsselmeer seas, a vast engineering feat that's the only route between the west of Holland and Friesland. It feels almost like the parting of the waves of Jordan, with the sea either side letting you through.

Later, offshore lights rock and sway as ships and boats are tossed on the waves; cars along the dam crash up skeins of water from the deluges as they proceed. I'm like a sea-beacon of light by the side of the road, wearing my newest reflectors and shining lights on the pack and adorning my coat. Drivers are courteous, lowering their headlight beams to spare me. I put my head down and run with a will.

I make it to Leewarden and, though sleepy and like a wet dog with my breath all steamy and hair like sodden fur, I feel so pleased. I'm warmly welcomed by Leewarden College students. Soon I feel great again thanks to them, dry the most essential items out, have a hot shower and rest. Then the real events of the day start. The roads become packed with runners, all wearing Rosie's Run T-shirts. We do 25km around sublime wooded Friesian countryside, with traditional homes with carved porches and a feeling all its own.

The support is such that I don't feel tired; the occasion ends with a concert by the local Shantykoor choir who sing great sea shanties and other songs. The words of 'Molly Malone' and 'Irish Eyes are Smiling' are still echoing in my head as I continue running towards Germany.

I head over the border on 2 November, one month since I've set off. I've now done 500 miles though the next 10,000 miles are going to be in kilometres, which is nice and encouraging. Kilometres may not be as lovable as miles (you never reach 'a kilometre-stone in life') but give the illusion of making progress by adding up more quickly.

I cross the border some distance beyond the last Dutch town of Groningham. No passport stamp, no officials. You'd hardly know you were in a different country. But I'm given a beautiful path beyond Bunde that will avoid all the busy roads.

The rain has started, everything keeps getting wet. I can't keep my eyes open all the same as the excitement of the last week is catching up. I'm so tired, I have to drop where I stop, which happens to be in the most beautiful late autumn forest. I'm never going to get over how I've always thought of Germany as an industrial country, yet it also has the most glorious broad-leaf forests I have ever seen. I prop up the bivvi, stuff myself into my great big double sleeping bag, and I'm gone, lost to the world.

One night I wake up in a terrible fright. Something has crashed into the bivvi. There's a loud squeal and heavy breathing outside. I say a lot of prayers all at once. I'm shaking all over, trying to gather my wits as I grab the torch.

CHAPTER 5

Eric the Wild Boar

Germany, November 2003

Something very alive, large, and struggling frantically, falls on top of me.

It's crazy trying to get the zip open, as everything is being flung all over the place. The bivvi hits a tree, and I get a thud on the head. I drop the torch, and am squashed flat in the dark. Luckily the torch is within my grasp.

I manage to get the strained zip open at last, and almost drop dead from astonishment. I'm still frightened but can't stop laughing either. Shaking almost as much as me and regarding me with little black short-sighted eyes, twitching his snout with fine whiskers and a pair of small tusks, is a wild boar. He seems quite young though large and appears to have collided with my home by accident. Probably out looking for truffles or something. He looks so sweet but I've heard that wild boars are dangerous. He's got himself caught up with the trotters in the guy rope, which on the bivvi are very low and he's twisting around until practically wearing the bivouac. We're both too squashed to move. I've heard that when dealing with bears, which I've never done before, you have to talk to them, so I say, 'It's OK, Eric —'

(the first name that comes to mind) '— I don't want any bacon for breakfast. Obelix might eat three wild boars for breakfast but not me!'

I'm so worried the bivvi will get wrecked, but he's standing stock still now although wound in it so tightly and it's all wedged around a tree root. I can hardly move either. It seems like hours have passed, though it's only moments since it all began. I never ever thought I'd end up being joined at the hip with a wild boar. Finally I sacrifice one of the guy ropes, cutting it with my small knife. Eric shakes himself free as if to see if he's really at liberty, then twists his little tail round and tears away with one last snort.

It's well after dawn. Sunshine comes through the golden leaves on the oak trees. Everything is drenched from the rain which has stopped without my noticing.

My tent is a scene of chaos but has somehow held together, although my precious Marmite and lavender oil have blended together, putting me off both for quite some time.

I'll never forget Eric the Wild Boar and the lesson he's taught me. This is a multifaceted journey, not just a run. In future I put little white ties on the guy-ropes to warn any short-sighted creatures that I'm there. Wild animals don't often attack you, but it doesn't pay to startle them. I'm to learn that they're not keen on a fight, as they don't wish to become injured themselves. There's not much joy in being an injured predator, because that way you don't get to eat. But I have to avoid another confrontation even like the one with berry- and truffle-eating Eric, however much we'd got along OK in the end, because the kit won't stand it.

I manage to gather my equipment together; it's pretty muddy and needs patching. I don't fancy sleeping in it before cleaning it up but I could do – it isn't too bad. I pack everything and have a good 35km run to Leer, the first German town. Ahead of me is the most beautiful sight: a hotel with pretty flower-boxes, the warmth and smell of hot coffee and signs for home-made apple strudel and delicious German sausages and sauerkraut.

I reach for the emergency pack of euros my brother Nicolas gave me before I left. The manager, dressed in black jacket and pin-striped trousers, grabs my soggy, muddy backpack as if it were Gucci luggage – only 40 euros with breakfast, he says. He dances me up the carpeted staircase, showing me into a room with a four-poster bed, pointing to the spacious gleaming bathroom, plucking a rose from a vase on the way up and flinging it into the washbasin, then leaves me to it. I'm so glad he doesn't reappear half an hour later. He'd never have recognised the place: my sleeping bags are hanging over plastic bags to catch the drops, with muddy leggings draped about the place. The great thing about hotel rooms is that the kit enjoys it as much as you do. I sink a small bottle of champagne that he's thoughtfully left beside the bed and fall fast asleep.

CHAPTER 6

Need Makes the Naked Lady Spin

Germany, November 2003

These are the foothills of the epic adventures ahead. I am in a hidden Germany I've never known existed: white-tailed deer leaping and bounding so high you'd think they had wings; cottages out of Hansel and Gretel; more hogs (though none behave like Eric); foxes and owls hunting at night, falcons and kestrels and hundreds of songbirds by day. As I nibble at black bread and cheese, the smaller birds often hop along with me, jumping on the crumbs.

I arrive at the historical town of Oldenburg among pretty buildings and churches with tall spires. I'd like to stay in Oldenburg one day with someone I love. I put the idea in a little bag inside my head called 'Later'. I hope it's a strong bag, as it holds a lot.

I think how lucky I've been to sleep beneath the beautiful stars in forests at night; to hear the wind stirring after a calm forest night; and get the smells and taste almost of the new day; the wild herbs, berries and fresh wild air – and to be on my way. The mornings are frosty and clear and everything just feels great.

I love these forests and towns that give me a feeling of running through a storybook. 'I'll be back, I keep telling myself.' On foot I am slow enough for the spell of my surroundings to catch and absorb me. They become part of me. Yet this is overshadowed by my emotions about the urgency of trying to keep going as well as I can. Russia lies ahead but it is at least 2,000 miles away.

I'm already on my third pair of shoes and they have looked after me really well, My legs feel fine. Top marathoners sometimes do 150 miles a week, just in training for a race, so the distance, even with the heavy pack, isn't so extreme as my pace is about 30–35km a day. If I think like this, the running is easier.

Over the next few days I cross footbridges over the huge autobahns or go through dark little tunnels leading beneath them, following mostly farm tracks and cycle paths. I'm so slow people often stop me to find out what I'm doing and give me valuable local directions. I am getting on reasonably well in German with the help of a phrase book, and going slowly makes me feel part of the communities I am running through, which makes me less lonely, and everybody is good to me. Some of the byways aren't on any map I've bought. I go north of Bremen after negotiating the bridge on the outskirts across the river, eventually reaching Buxthude and I'm 20km from Hamburg where I need to collect a parcel.

I'm given keys to a closed campsite so I can shower in the toilet block. The showers work but the lights are dim and while I'm showering I hear crunching beneath my feet and realise the floor's full of broken glass, as one of the windows has been smashed by the winter storms. I spend a long time picking it out of my feet but think no more of it.

I arrive in Hamburg at last on 11 November, and find a policeman leaning against his motorcycle as I reach the city centre after hours of heading in from the outskirts. He signs my logbook with a flourish, directing me to the Allianz Cornhill building – a glittering skyscraper. One of the most difficult things on this run is getting an address where I can get my kit sent ahead. Geoff Hall who works for Allianz Cornhill in London has arranged for their office in Hamburg to kindly help and receive a box of equipment for me which has arrived. Myrto Reiger and her colleagues greet me cheerfully, dragging in what they call 'the Rosie Parcel'.

I check out the website which is going so well. I'm inspired all the time by the way people have been helping non-stop; most of all, the heart-warming and exceptional support from my 'A Team' back at home who have been in on it from day one. This sustained assistance is so valuable. Ann has even sent a 'Red Cross parcel' she's made up for me, containing fruitcake and home-made apple pie, that's somehow survived. The items need to be packed into my ruck-sack. They all help, as the poor pack grows and grows. Cakes and coffee are served, and they produce a gift of a big box of chocolates, sharing my joy as I open letters from family and hand around photos. I get out all the treats, letters from my family, vital winter kit from PHD and new shoes. It's like a birthday party! I leave a couple of hours later feeling happy and exuberant.

The first place I arrive at that has rooms is a very prosperous bordello, one of the best in town, says the landlady as she shows me up the stairs. They have plenty of rooms for the budget traveller as well. The whole establishment seems to have been designed as a stage set for a Feydeau farce – with separate staircases so those going up for fun won't collide with those coming down and be embarrassed, she informs me archly, taking me up to my tiny room.

It's only when I stop and the euphoria of arrival wears off that I become aware of the extreme pain in my left foot. I sink on the bed, close the gingham curtains and examine my foot which had trodden on the glass and which is now very painful. There's a huge lump like a corn with a glistening sliver of glass still in it and the callous has grown around it. I get out my small knife and dig the glass out a bit ferociously, but it doesn't work and the foot soon becomes agonising. The little room is spotless but black mice keep darting here and there. If I turn on the light, I even find them sitting on the shelf. So there is wildlife here too. They entertain me all through the night as I can't sleep.

Next day a nearby pharmacy gives me the name of a doctor. I call Ann in Tenby, still keeping an eye on my finances, and go for it. The nurse wraps a black band with a blood-pressure measuring dial around my left ankle and injects my foot. The doctor proceeds to cut off most of my third toe but it's probably just the skin. The nurse wraps it all up in thick bandages so it resembles a Yeti's foot and says I have to buy a giant blue surgical slipper she's produced.

No running for two weeks, the doctor says.

I retire to my bordello, determined to make it in three days. The foot will heal fast as I'm fit. I'm concerned that I had a visa for the little piece of Russia called Kallingrad, which is all on its own in Europe; an extra visa to get through this area has also been arranged by Liza but will run out if I don't get there soon enough.

I get ready. It's 12 November; if I can leave on the 14th, that would be fantastic. Behind my hotel, alternating with the many wild-looking clip joints and naked shows, are small, inexpensive shops selling food from around the world, ranging from African sweet yams to delicious tiny Caribbean bananas and rye-bread.

The kiosk walls in the many small businesses offering cheap phone-calls are paper-thin. As I queue up with others, mostly from a large, hard-working immigrant community living quietly alongside the thriving nightlife, I recognise joy in the voices at once as soon as anyone gets through.

It's the first time on my run I've been amongst others far from their homes who have left families behind in more straitened circumstances of poverty and war than I could ever dream. They are sweet people and very polite to me. We communicate with words and gestures. As an Icelandic friend later tells me, 'Need makes the naked lady spin.'

The mice look on with definite approval as I unpack my purchases of figs, dates, cheese and bread until I shut the whole lot into a tin with a firm lid.

I call Eve and James, and the line is so clear I feel I am reaching out and hugging them. They are part of me – the very best part – and I feel so close to them. I am happy and cheered knowing that everything is well at home. As many parents with grown-up families do, I feel that Eve and James and Pete are more than daughter and son and son-in-law to me; they are friends who I admire so much as well as love. They are in their thirties and with their own lives, but they are so good to me. They live far from Tenby, and often in the past we've been at the end of a phone like now. The difference this time is both that I shall be gone so long; but also that we are perhaps getting even closer in spirit than ever before.

It's a delightful boost when Geoff flies to Hamburg to walk with me for several kilometres before catching his flight back the same day. He also takes some good photos for the sponsors, which has been hard for me to achieve alone.

As we set off, I find that I can cope without too much trouble with the bad foot. I wear a running shoe on one foot, surgical slipper on the other. With a plastic bag over the bandage, it works OK. Every time I get tired we call into a shop; they pull out a chair so I can rest for a few minutes but I soon get stronger.

The only sad thing on the way from Hamburg is that Tenby Bear gets lost. I feel more than a twinge of sorrow. He's been firmly tied and squashed into the backpack, but has vanished. Maybe he didn't approve of the Red Light District or, on the contrary, liked it too much and has rushed back there to join in the fun. I hope some child in Hamburg who needs a beautiful bear will find him and love him a lot.

* * *

By 15 November I've made 14km. I'm out in the forests again, it's nearly −8 and the trees look like gossamer with stars caught in the frost branches. It always turns me inside-out with feelings I can't describe, because of the sheer beauty and the feeling of being all alone in it.

It's cold but doesn't rain, which is lucky as the foot stays dry and doesn't get infected. I'm gradually able to wear a shoe on my bad foot, though without an insole.

By 17 November I've reached Ratzeburg. Between here and Gadebusch, I run across the former border of East Germany. There is more difference between the old East Germany and West Germany than I realised. Bus stops in villages don't have shelters, there are fewer cycle tracks. Houses are older, usually having smaller windows; penny marts and stalls sell everything. They seem quietly spoken, private folk who smile a bit when they hear my efforts at German. I had to learn the basics of five different languages before leaving home because in many cases nobody outside towns can speak English. It also seems to be a courtesy as well as necessity to learn a bit of each language.

In a penny mart I meet Marion, selling salami with her husband. She writes in my book and says she'd love to cycle across Africa one day. 'A dream is as necessary as being able to eat. It's even more important when it's all you have,' she says. 'We'll go one day. Don't tell my husband yet as it's a secret.' I can see he knows, from the affectionate smile he gives her. Maybe they should get a tandem, but then again maybe not. A week ago near Hamburg on a cycle path I saw a couple on a tandem. The man in front was beaming, pedalling fast. Luckily he couldn't look back to see his wife her face like thunder, and not pedalling at all.

Chunks of snow decorate the sweet-smelling pine forest after the first snowfall. Beneath mighty trees, little spruces and firs, delicately fringed with snow, are waiting to be collected to give pleasure over Christmas. I think, *I want one like this next Christmas*. I imagine my family sitting around it; parcels beneath. I think, *It's what I have always taken for granted that means the most now*. That's the biggest lesson of my run so far.

People show me paths from farm to farm and through mighty pine woods before I head back onto a big road leading to Schwerin with its Cinderella-like castle. The last big place was Hamburg. I'm finding that reaching a town becomes part of the adventure.

My foot is much better. The rest and recent low mileage have helped too – I ran 46km today to get to Schwerin, but am pretty tired; I decide, it's definitely time for a treat.

The first hotel I call at is expensive; the elderly blonde woman has a mean mouth. But a handsome young man with flowing hair is in charge of the next. He has a little dog with a bow in its hair that never leaves his heels. He welcomes me and charges half price. I have dinner in a hotel cafe with large aquaria everywhere, so one is truly dining with the fish; there are no other human guests. I retire to a comfy room where I can sort everything out and have a bath, soak the sore foot – and stretch in the warm water and luxuriate deliciously.

Next morning I run in lashing rain across the Rampamoor, leading past mangroves and swamps close to the road between the water. It's said to be a famous beauty spot but is ghoulish and full of restless ghosts as I cross in a near gale.

A downpour has caused splashes of rainwater to be released in the trees. Each time the branches shake it's like living under a waterfall so I have to keep moving the bivvi in the middle of the night. Since by now there's no chance of getting to sleep, I do some writing. As my handwriting is a trainee MI5's operative's masterclass in decoding, especially by the flickering torchlight, I have to find new batteries. The bivvi suddenly seems larger once everything is brighter and now I can read what I have written I'm wondering why I bothered in the first place.

I arrive at a strange place in the woods. A sign says it's Raststate Rosenhof. The door's unlocked so I push it. There are tree branches inside decorating it, so it still seems like part of the forest. There's nobody there. Places are laid out with bowls and spoons, as in Goldilocks and the Three Bears. I shout out 'Hello'. A bouncy-looking man with gleaming eyes and a jolly expression appears, introducing himself as Jurgen. He treats me to coffee and produces a tray of freckled eggs in front of my eyes, carrying them off to the kitchen and personally cooking me a delicious breakfast: eggs, bacon and sausage, better than Goldilocks' porridge. It stops raining and I get going. A car comes roaring up behind me on the country road. It's Jurgen. As it's early in the morning he's dug his wife out of bed to meet up with me. He's wrapped a blanket around her and brought her curlers and all.

They have come because his parents have both died of cancer. They embrace me and wish me 'gut speed'. The warmth with which they say it keeps me going a long way.

Bruel is desolate and very windy when I get there. I wash my thermal vest in the Ladies (*Damen*) in one of the cafes, put it on wet as usual to be dried by my body – I'm my own clothes-horse. Drying is helped by the blast of the slipstream of passing juggernauts. The only problem is I haven't rinsed the apple shampoo out of my clothes so everything smells of apple. Talk about 'Cider with Rosie'.

It often occurs to me that running as a way of travelling is a mixture of practical things, myths and unspoken laws:

- Say thank you to the ground you have slept on.
- Pick up any litter as if it's 50 euro notes.
- Never miss the chance to be happy.

I'll never get over the feeling of climbing a hill and seeing the red roof of the first house in the next village. In this case it's Grobraden, where there's an old Slavonic castle. There are two languages, just like in Wales, and the history goes back thousands of years.

I carry on over the next 150km to Usedom, a historical spot with a thin strip of land binding the Acterwasser or lake along the road that runs to Poland. I am tempted to stay longer in Usedom. There are breathtaking old oaks and beech trees among frosty, feathered pine trees. I see a sign beside a footpath saying there are wolves here, but don't see any. There are no campsites open so I stay in the woods, tidily and quietly.

Lying awake listening to the noises of the night when most humans are asleep, I think nobody on earth knows

where I'm sleeping tonight except the owls and silent creatures who may be watching and the little black beetles that
become rainbow-coloured when you shine the torch on
them. I'll always remember Usedom for its tranquillity and
wildlife.

From here, on 1 December, I cross the border to Poland.

CHAPTER 7

Rip Van Winkle in a Snow-hole

Poland, December 2003

Everything is black. There's a crushing weight on top of me. I've gone to sleep with the torch in my hand, and flicker it on to see the inside of the bivvi filled with a huge tangle of frayed rope.

It's not rope at all. It's actually my half-frozen breath that's been recycled, melted and refrozen, as there's so little air. I grab the zip and have to force it open. A heap of snow comes in and mixes with my frozen breath. I burrow and dig my way up.

The full moon is shining down on a totally white landscape and I'm in a snowdrift, 5ft deep. Again! The stars gleam into my snow-hole. Inside the bivvi, the sleeping bags and saucepans are covered with ice, my black bag with precious items has turned into a white bag. I can't believe I just camped here last night. It's as if I've been here for a thousand years and I'm Rip Van Winkle who went to sleep in a cave for 1000 years.

I make the hole larger into a kind of cave, then get the stove out. I had it in the sleeping bag to keep warm as I've been having trouble lighting it. I stick the lighter down my front inside my clothes to warm up a bit too and lose it for ever. Luckily, I've got waterproofed matches in a tin. I chip ice from the saucepan, triumphantly making snowy porridge for breakfast.

When the stove won't go I spoon coffee powder into the mug, topping it up with cold water, thinking of it as Starbucks. It isn't bad – great training for the imagination.

Most things have to be done differently – most important, the chamber-pot. In eighteenth-century England even the grandest homes had potties under the beds. Nobody wished to walk down icy corridors in search of facilities in the middle of night. My pot is more of a mountaineer's emergency pee tin, but has a good lid, which is its most important feature. I *can't* wriggle out into the darkness and snow at –15°C, freeze my bottom and bring all the snow in with me.

Vivid human encounter and deep solitude alternate like movements in a symphony. I love Poland. After the loneliness I find the people are so warm and full of fun, with the laughter and spirit of those who have known harsh times throughout their history but have never been conquered inside themselves.

There were two days of golden autumn just before the blizzard. These last moments seemed brighter and stronger as if to give a memory for the winter that wouldn't fail during the months ahead.

The wind flying in ebullient little whirlwinds makes a merry-go-round of golden leaves. The last colours before the snows come are blazing scarlet, crimson and orange in the forests. The last dance of the leaves.

The first town I reach, Swinouscie, is an Aladdin's cave of markets, an extravaganza of life and colour. Hot-water bottles dangle above stalls in their dozens, top of the range in the colder weather, along with thick socks, batteries of all sizes, spicy-smelling sausages, vegetables brightly displayed, exquisitely etched glassware. People hug each other, laugh a lot, wear big furry hats. My heart is lifted by hundreds of beautiful little horses pulling taxi carriages at a canter, with bells jingling merrily, or standing with faces deep in fat nosebags. I've fallen for a bright bay pony with a wild black mane and four white socks.

I'm patting the horse when his owner comes up, a white-haired energetic old man. He gets out his accordion and sings me a song. I don't understand the lyrics, but it sounds great. I haven't expected to arrive in Poland and be sere-naded. I'm huge in damp coats and think my face is muddy from the lorries coming through the customs. The next thing he does is to get out a big clean white hanky, reach out and tenderly wipe my face. He then declares I have to marry him, he needs a wife and apparently I'm just right. I think he's only asking me to make me smile, as I'm cold and lonely, but it does cheer me up. I imagine it's typical Polish gallantry. He speaks in English but can't understand anything I say to him. I'll always remember the first words I string together in Polish with the help of the phrasebook: 'Thank you very, very much, but I'm *spoken for.*'

He kisses my hand and vanishes. He'd mentioned he was nearly 90, hard to believe, and glad to be still working. I never discover his name, but he's wonderful and leaves me feeling all made up.

I head off across the Wolin, practically an island linked by a tiny strip of land and bridge at a place called Dziwinów to the west of the north coast. There's a spectacular nature reserve with majestic forests. The snows begin hitting hard. Deep winter arrives overnight. The holiday village buildings and campsites along the coast are ghosts. Buildings roar and shake in the blizzards. Doors to tourist cafes with tantalising signs for ice-cream and hot coffee are locked and barred, but the local farming community hang out in occasional cafes. I'm able to take off the wet kit discreetly and wring out my socks and vests. Nobody asks me to leave, even though I'm making puddles on the floors. Of course, the proprietors and customers are brilliant to me, as they have to be out themselves tending the farms. I buy pickles, black bread, wonderful sausage full of calories, and am fed hot beer – the locals say it's the finest cure for the cold and everything else too.

I'm managing in Polish because of their huge efforts to encourage me, as few people in the countryside speak English. It gets to me so much that in the small, struggling communities, in cafes and markets, people seem to understand what I'm doing, 'this crazy marathon', and why: the outer and inner journey, the purpose of it, without too many words.

Cancer is a problem here too. I learn there's a lot of it along the Polish coast. In Kosalin, someone calls the local paper and I do a stumbling interview in Polish to promote cancer awareness and health checks. I am so pleased that my message might reach someone here and help them. I think of Clive, still wondering how it would have turned out if we'd gone to the doctor earlier. The reasons for my run are not left behind. If you do something for a reason, I'm discovering, the reason itself gives back the help ten thousandfold, because it makes you so much more determined.

CHAPTER 8

Touching the Stars

Poland, December 2003

It's −20°C but a fine morning on 9 December. I am too ambitious doing my washing in the cold of the woods. My socks feel like they're beginning to run around the world by themselves so I take the chance of washing them in water I've melted from snow. Not to waste water, and feeling proud of my frugality, I try washing my hair which is dank, half-frozen and sticky with frozen sweat. The ends sticking out under my muddy balaclava have become ingrained with dirt from passing lorries flinging up grubby snow over me along slushy, icy roads. What a mistake. My hair is frozen before I'm able to get the soap out and stands on end so I look like a punk rocker with icicles for earrings. When I get back to my socks they have frozen solid. I left them tied onto the outside of my pack, forgetting I can never dry things this way when it's icy. They are so hard, I have to break them apart.

Undeterred I run into Slupsk and become lured by the lights of Restaurcja McDonald's gleaming through the blowing snow. Eating spaghetti, cooked in snow-water with bits of grit in it, makes you a fan of McDonald's. Especially as I've learned they started the Ronald McDonald Houses, enabling parents of seriously sick children to stay near them when they're in hospital. The restaurants serve budget salads and yogurts with fruit. You don't have to eat burgers and chips unless you want to.

The Slupsk McDonald's manager and staff, cheery-looking in their red shirts, seem to be students working their way through college. Instead of being disapproving at the spectacle of a muddy, snowy, dripping person large with giant backpack, they enthusiastically give permission for me to use their washroom. It all brings back memories of McDonald's in Lancashire, and my training in the art of making do before setting off. At least I don't get my head stuck between the basin and the taps this time – and the hot water is bliss.

Yet treats like this aren't going to save me. Security can only come from being vulnerable out there in the forests, and learning how to deal with it. I have to sleep out most nights because of budget and distances between places, training myself to think of my bivvi not as McDonald's but a tiny Hotel Sheraton. It *has* to have everything I need because cafes and other safety nets will get scarce from now on. As days shorten and conditions harden, the only way to do the miles is on a sort of 24-hour clock. Running a few hours, then stopping and resting and getting going again, like being on- and off-watch at sea or shiftwork. So the bivvi is very convenient. Curl up, sleep and go. The ability to be able to rest along the road makes the hitches in doing this well worth overcoming.

Simple things and high-tech items work together. A pencil is essential for notes because it writes long after the ink in pens and biros has frozen. Vaseline is good for protecting skin, especially on my feet. I have a tiny purple spot of mild frostbite on one toe. This happened the one morning I forgot the Vaseline. My feet also got really cold when I tried running in boots and couldn't dry the frozen sweat out of them. I'm much more comfortable in my Saucony running shoes especially when I adapt them for the freezing conditions. I line them with rabbit fur and weatherproof them with a spray. They're light enough to run in, don't give me blisters and can be dried in the sleeping bag at night.

I get into the habit of heating water and putting it in a drinking bottle and at night wrapping socks around the hot-water bottle or pulling them over it. Unlike rubber hot-water bottles, it's exactly the right shape for socks, and can also be put inside my shoes to warm them before I put them on, which is a delicious feeling.

The finest help of all is the state-of-the-art quality of the bivouac itself, and the brilliant feather down and Gortex clothing and sleeping-bag system. Sir Ranulph Fiennes and other great explorers always depend on Peter Hutchinson's PHD and Terra Nova, and I'm so lucky to have them. Because I can only carry the bivvi and not a mountain tent, due to the weight factor, Peter has designed the clothing and bags especially, knowing that snow and ice will be part of my life, and that the ice will often melt and refreeze. The scene in my bivvi often looks so terrible that it's unimaginable a human could live in there, but it's fine. It just requires another way of thinking and it works because of the kit. I have more feathers than a falcon. The outer layers are cold and icy or damp, but the inner layers of down feathers, like those of birds, are always dry, and my skin is warm. My core body heat is stable and good.

My training descends into pure decadence when I reach Gdansk on 13 December 2003. A Rosie Parcel has been sent to Allianz Polsa. The staff even open on a stormy Sunday to welcome me and give me my box. Although for years Chief Investment Officer with Allianz Cornhill, Geoff's frame of mind is just like when he was a student and needed to learn to drive six different types of bus to qualify for a job with public transport in Australia. When Geoff says he'll help he means it: he's a runner and cares that I succeed.

Somehow, the vital new equipment is crammed into the backpack, including the big extra sleeping bag for the next harsh stage: shoes; some stores; and weatherproof leggings. The backpack is nearly bursting with its contents, now weighing 23kg.

That evening the director's assistant Isabella and her boyfriend Darek take me off to a fabulous Russian restaurant in town to be plied with caviar and fresh fish from the bay, washed down with Polish vodka and blackcurrant juice. Darek says it's only 'vodka sparring' as Polish vodka is not as strong as Russian. 'Just training,' he adds. It's very energising, but I've never slept so soundly. I curl up on the sofa of their comfy flat, cuddled up to and watched over by their beautiful black dog Myrto. You can tell what people are like by the happiness of their animals.

I'm in the wilds for most of the two weeks up to Christmas on my way to the Lithuanian border. This section of the journey becomes strange and metaphysical. I feel my family walking with me, so strongly that I believe if I turn around in dark forests I'll see them. And I do, more clearly than when we'd been together. It will be my grandson Michael's second birthday on 19 December. I'm excited for Michael, yet sad at the time I have lost with him. He is so wonderful and all I want to do is hug him. I charge the satphone specially so I can sing him Happy Birthday.

Two days before Christmas, near the Lithuanian border, I lie with my head out of the bivvi, wrapped in my thickest coat and with the hood drawn tightly. It's such a beautiful clear moonlit night. I can see thousands of Christmas trees.

Starlight tumbles like shiny crystals over the dark majestic firs and silver birch trees. I gaze at the sky above the forest clearing. Sirius is bright and I can see Orion's Belt and a million others. I name the stars after my family – Eve, Peter, James, Michael, Marianne and all the people I love. I think about all the worlds out there, shining down to earth with all their strength. They are all so far away that time hardly seems to matter any more. All that ever happened is here, part of now, giving me strength. Soon I'll be home, I say to myself. Time is a friend after all. I'm touching the stars, yet I'm closer to home than those stars are to me.

CHAPTER 9

A Stranger is Family

Poland, December 2003

In Poland it's the custom to set an extra place at Christmas
for 'The Unknown Guest'. It's early morning on Christmas
Eve when I find out how true this is. I've run through a
snowstorm and gale that's just eased back when I see a
diminutive figure rushing after me, whipping up a whirlwind of snow. Following her is a little girl with snowflakes
in her curls sticking out from her woolly hat and a small dog
with wagging tail, chugging through the snow like a miniature snowplough, his legs too short to leap over the drifts.

'*Nesoey Sisiat!*' she shouts. '*Happy Christmas!*' Unlike most
people in this area, she speaks perfect English. Dorota,
daughter Kasia, aged eight, and their sweet little dog Eny
lead me to their home a short distance away in Budry. I
follow them with pleasure but it's like a force of absolute will.
They apparently feel they have to spoil me. They haven't
even known I'm coming, but spotted me in the distance.

'Nobody should be alone at Christmas,' says Dorota.

The building is a tall ex-communist warren of small
apartments. The exterior is grey, brutally functional, like the
communist buildings surviving in Germany, Albania and

Romania which I saw on a previous journey. But inside it's very different: Polish candles of hope and for the spirit of Christmas are on the shelves and tables. There's the smell of warm baking. Sweet-smelling fir branches, bells and tinsel decorate the living room for the festive season; sprigs of fir hang over bookshelves filled with books in Polish and English. They even have *The Pickwick Papers* and *Oliver Twist*.

They want me to stay for Christmas Day. Christmas is traditionally a closed circle yet a stranger like me is given such affection and welcome. 'A stranger is never a stranger,' she says. 'A stranger *is* family.' I feel so moved yet I also need to be back on the road.

So they deluge me with a Christmas Eve I'll never forget, putting music on and feeding me with carp her friends caught. It's deliciously baked and, I learn, the traditional Christmas meal in this part of Poland. We also eat Moczka, a sweet pudding tasting of poppy seeds, nuts and fruit. Dorota has a computer and sends the first message to the website that James has had for a while. I also write an email to James and Eve. I couldn't have asked for a lovelier Christmas gift. Before I leave, Kasia ties tinsel to my backpack, 'To bring you happiness and luck,' she says. They heap me with delicious food before hugging me and saying goodbye.

There is a party after all, because the magpies and starlings are fascinated by Kasia's tinsel and keep appearing, looking for a chance to steal it. The cake-crumbs make the sparrows and finches even more eager to follow my trail than usual, as the fare is so fancy. They're still Clive's 'little feathered hooligans'.

*　*　*

It's 30km to the next town, Goldup, the only big place in this area. I've made good progress and find myself running through the hustle and bustle and last-minute shoppers. I'm concerned about my budget as always, and don't feel like staying in a hotel at Christmas anyway. I run on until I reach beautiful woods and camp in a wide clearing.

I sleep soundly, waking early on Christmas Day. It's a cold morning, −21°C, but the air is fresh and clear. I'm warmly dressed and a pale band of gold around the edge of the sky leads me on. I get up and run. For some reason, I feel must keep going, keep running on this special day, though I don't know why …

I haven't got far when a car draws up and a middle-aged couple get out. They stop especially to talk, looking downcast. They speak French which I can speak, saying something about having been looking and searching for a sign. They hug me, seeming overwhelmed to see me. They want to give me their email address. After they drive off I see they have written in my book: 'Our son Guillamine took his life on 30 October 2003 to join his great father in the sky. You have appeared to us as a marvellous star and a message of love. You have given us hope.'

It's hard to write about this. I cry and cry, which is something I never do. I don't really know why they have said I've given them hope. If so, I'm so glad. I cheer up at the thought of action and decide to run for Guillamine through Christmas, to think about this man whom I haven't met and can never meet, and about his parents Christian and Elizbieta. I do believe thinking about someone can help. Thoughts and prayers are powerful messengers. These two have touched my life and given me more courage. The to-ing and fro-ing between feeling my family are with me and the loneliness that cuts like a knife has gone. Perhaps because it makes me realise I have so much.

Next day I reach Dubeniniki and meet a wonderful lady called Bozenna. 'You must come home for a meal,' she greets me, 'but first we go to church.' The huge church is packed, people standing shoulder to shoulder. The singing is powerful and stirring, every voice from the thronged masses joining in. There are guitars and children singing and the christening of a three-week-old baby at the end of it all.

It has been my policy not to cross a border late at night, because I'd be in a new country and not sure how to handle everything. I sleep this side of the Lithuanian border beneath trees all bowed and broken under the weight of the snow. One tree is creaking, but I can't tell which one and I'm so tired I don't move. I hope it won't fall on me, and that everything is all right.

CHAPTER 10

The World of Special So-called Ordinary People

Lithuania, January 2004

Girls with high cheekbones and hair dyed bright scarlet or green. Houses leaning sideways, after years of being buffeted by storms; firs bowed by ice, gales like moonstorms and people so full of life that young and old they seem to be dancing as they proceed along the hazardous icy pavements in the little towns. These are my first impressions of Lithuania.

Life beneath the razzmatazz seems hard. As in Poland, everybody here seems to have a passionate determination that they won't get bowed down like the trees in the storms. I run along a road parallel to the highway to reach the first town Marijampole, 19km north of the Polish border. I continue on many small roads leading north, though more snowed in every day. On New Year's Eve I'm invited in by a charming family who I meet at a little village store near Kazlu Ruda. They are Lena, who is Russian; Artur, a Lithuanian; Elzbieta and Ivan, their children; and Babai the cat. The apartment has no doors. I think they're too busy to put them up as they both have three jobs. A teacher only earns the equivalent of US$30 a month. Lena looks like a ballet dancer. She's tall, slim and very beautiful with long hair and seems to prance and whirl instead of just walking around. The most precious object in her apartment is the washing machine her husband bought after being away on a contracting job. There are presents and extra celebration, Lena explains, because Artur has just been paid for the first time for a year as his employer needed to keep his workers' wages to stay in business.

Lena is imitated by her three-year-old daughter, who's been given rollerblades and is trying out the prancing on her skates. She keeps falling over, but laughs and gets up again, going for longer every time. It's happy chaos and much fun. The cat leaps out of the way as if wishing it had rollerskates too and is practising quick escapes in the small living room that doubles as a bedroom. Lena empties my pack, putting clothes, that still seem to have bits of the forest from several different countries in them, into the wash. The washing itself is like a fiesta. Then Lena grabs some salts she says are great for the feet and flings them into the bath, a rare boon. There's no door here either. For modesty's sake she hangs up a blanket and throws me some of her clothes to wear, so I can get mine off for the wash.

After that we eat and eat. I'm so glad I bought sausage, cakes and chocolates at the little village store, but it isn't much compared to what they give me to feast on. We watch the New Year celebrations on Lithuanian TV. Artur says that despite the show of optimism on TV, getting work is tough now. It's not easy to get a visa to travel in most of Europe, and also they're now required to have a visa for Russia, which they used not to need. They are proud that Lithuania in 1991 was the first country to become independent among the former Soviet republics, after much bloodshed through the years, but they also feel hemmed in, in a new kind of way.

As midnight approaches, we head gaily out with all the others pouring from apartments blocks, to see in the New Year. Lots of singing, and fireworks blaze their path beneath the crescent moon.

There is a dangerous river beyond here. I'm grateful to a man from the next village who tells me the river Nemunas has no ferries in winter, but that the ice isn't yet strong enough to walk across on. I'm saved a long stretch of retracing steps. I go instead via a little place called Geariliavi. It's cold, but I take my mind off it by eating Lena's pasties that she's packed in profusion to keep me going.

I sink up to the waist in snow. It doesn't get ploughed here. The wind's howling and by evening the bivvi is frozen so hard rolled up in the pack that it's all stuck together. I'm frightened that I can't prise the opening apart enough to climb in it to get shelter. It's painful and slow to break it open but I manage to get inside. It becomes an oddly shaped frozen igloo, smaller than ever as it has contracted and iced together. I have to take everything to bed with me, especially the shoes. It's not enough to bring them inside the bivvi. They freeze so hard I can't undo the laces and get my feet in.

I try bypassing Kaunas, as the main road through is full of lorries flinging snow and slush over me, but I get lost, eventually finding myself in the centre of the city after midnight, and carry on into the side-streets. Everything is dark and seems asleep. A hotel I pass looks expensive, its door locked

for the night. I'm walking, not running – actually I'm creep-
ing along very tired with head bowed, when I almost collide
with a wheelchair that has fallen over.

A man is still in it. He's crying but nobody has heard. He
seems scared when he sees me. He can't right the wheelchair
as he has no legs. He just lies wrapped in rags, clutching the
chair and trying to stay in it as he lies sideways on the snow.
He's trying to gather some coins that have spilt from a small
cardboard collecting box. I'm not frightened of him; he's the
frightened one. He shrinks from me. He takes hold of my
bright torch and shines it at me. I can only see his eyes, a small
part of his face, as he has a large scarf, but his eyes are gentle.
I definitely know that he's not intending me harm; indeed
he's frightened I might attack or rob him. Then he suddenly
smiles, even though his thin face and scraggy beard are still
trembling with cold, or fear or emotion. He keeps looking at
me as if I'm not real. It's a massive struggle to push the wheelchair upright while he's still in it. If he came out of it, neither
of us would manage. He starts talking and I get out my
dictionary. Certainly he doesn't wish to go hospital, he tries to
tell me, but he does have a place to go, or so it seems with the
help of the phrasebook and signs he makes.

Down those awful empty dark streets I push him, as
through the labyrinths of hell. It's very hard to push small
rusty wheels through the snow. I don't know how he usually
does it. Eventually, he points this way and that, and we come
to a part of town where people are still out drinking and
eating at a small cafe.

The café manageress, like someone from the movies,
broad and glamorous in big shawls and necklaces, clasps my

hands and thanks me for bringing him as he's been lost. I soon understand that the man I've brought in is a war hero known as Vladimir who's fallen on hard times. Vladimir is taken off to the washroom by friends to clean up after the fall. A crowd of girls looking pretty and warm, mostly dressed in silver miniskirts and practical thick leggings like dancers wear, throng around him, kissing him, saying things like, 'Don't be long. Your drink's waiting for you.' They laugh, telling me they love him. He's their grandfather. I'm given a hot drink and sausage and soup. Some of the people stay around the cafe all night as they too have nowhere to go. The manager shows me a sofa in a side room where I can sleep. I want to sleep dreaming of all the faces, all the hollow-eyed office workers who've never got home, tramps, factory shift-workers and women who invite me to take their photos so I could send them a husband from England.

People with nothing want to help me in every way. I don't need any help, but they do. So, it continues while I'm in Lithuania. I learn about the brave, tragic Lithuanian history, and understand for the first time that the run around the world is going to be more full of surprises and unforgettable sharp lessons than I'd ever thought; that most memorable of all will not be the dangers, the cold, the encounters with death that lie ahead, but the fact that it's a living circle of testimony to community and humanity, and that there *is* a united world. The world of special so-called ordinary people.

CHAPTER 11

Shaken not Stirred

Latvia, January 2004

By contrast with the cosy cafe, on Sunday, 4 January in the woods, I'm eating oatmeal with snow. It's an awful breakfast but my stove has been broken for three weeks and I can't make any hot meals or drinks. I've arranged to collect a new one in Riga which is now only 210km away. I can't wait. Luckily I'm on a main E64 highway heading up by way of Panevezys towards the Latvian border, as the secondary roads are closed and six foot deep in snow. I can get meals now and again at the Lucoil Service Stations; otherwise it's bread and cheese and muesli.

The damage to the bivvi started by Eric the Wild Boar has also got worse and the zip has finally given way. I'm getting a new bivvi sent with my stove but in the meantime I have to wedge the flap shut by leaning my backpack against it. This works fine as the flap is always frozen stiff as a board and stays steady.

Psychologically, the fact that I can manage in a damaged bivvi and without a stove at −20°C is reassuring. I am getting hardier and I feel more confident I'll manage when the temperatures start dropping to −30°C. Even so, at the end of the day I almost always just drop in my tracks wherever I stop. I have no spare energy to run extra kilometres to find a town and accommodation. It's better for my budget too.

I run under a bright icy moon with dark woods and mountains of snow either side of the road; lorries throw heaps of slush over me, but the backpack cover is good and I hardly care any more. There's nothing I can do about it. I'm used to getting grubby.

I get very excited as I approach the Latvian border on 9 January. Another country. The furry-hatted customs officers wave me through and are most polite. I'm pleased I came this way.

Next morning a big black official-looking car draws up alongside me as I'm running along and three good-looking men climb out like something out of James Bond. They shake my hand, greeting me warmly. It's a big surprise.

'Are you Welsh?' one asks.

They are Brian Court, UK Adviser to the Lithuanian Ministry of Defence; Lieutenant Colonel Mike Clements, UK Defence Attaché in Lithuania; Paul Hutton, Assistant Attaché; and Rokas Boreiko their Lithuanian Defence Section Driver.

They stand in the snow chatting, apparently impervious to the weather. Despite their smart greatcoats, I fear they're cold, as I'm wearing three down jackets. This amuses them and they remark that it's me they're concerned about. They have been listening to the news on their radio, it's −15°C with windchill, and −22 not far away on the Belarus border, but they say I look as if I'm coping. They're the first British people I've met for over six weeks. I can't stop smiling and talking nineteen to the dozen. It's the first time I've spoken English for so long. Yet I feel choked up with emotion at the same time.

They lend me their satphone because communication has been tremendously hard recently. It's brilliant to get through to Eve and hear that all's OK back home. As always Eve and Jim are here with me all the time. As Patty Agostinelli, a wonderful friend I meet later on the run, beautifully puts it, 'A family is a village. You're close wherever you are, anywhere in the world.'

I think we're getting closer while I'm running, because we share and send powerful thoughts. This is on my mind all the time. Chatting with Eve lightens my heart, brightens the day. I give the diplomats back their phone with all my thanks. Brian Court generously gives me some Latvian currency, as 'a contingency fund' as he calls it, and says they'll let the consul in Riga know I'm on my way.

They've made my day. Later, they write a graphic email to James for the website:

We were driving south, approximately 64km from Riga, back to the British Embassy in Lithuania. Almost unnoticed, we flashed past a diminutive figure wrapped against the biting weather and burdened by a large red rucksack, running north to Riga. My colleague, Paul Hutton, said, 'Do you suppose that is the Welsh lady running around the world for charity? We started looking for a support team, but there was no evidence of any. We drove on for a few miles speculating and when our curiosity got the better of us, Rokas our driver did an about-turn at a convenient roundabout and hunted her down. I wound down the window and asked, feeling rather foolish, 'Are you Welsh?' The mystery runner pulled back her hood, took off her sunglasses and mittens, gave us a huge smile, and confirmed that she was indeed Rosie Swale Pope.

I run to the town of Jecava, stopping at Cafe Balta Roze to fix a wobbling filling with Krazy Glue, said to be great for this purpose by a lady in charge of a small shop. She speaks English too, which appears to be more usual in Latvia than in many places I've been. For a few minutes it seems just the job. But the glue makes my eyes water. Not sure it's going to be a tremendous success.

I sneeze and the tooth crown shoots out, to my huge embarrassment nearly hitting an old gentleman quietly drinking his coffee at the next table. He politely picks up the little glistening white and broken tooth, wraps it in tissue and gravely hands it back to me with a bow. The manageress tells me he's worried it will be expensive for me if I lose it. Then I'm on my way again.

The last 50km to Riga take me through stretches of mighty forests that cover half of Latvia. The only bare patches have some of Latvia's numerous lakes deep beneath them, under four or five foot of snow and ice. There's no secrets in the snow. I see the tracks of deer and paw-marks and the hopping and skipping tracks that have no beginning, no end, that belong to birds who have a little walk or scamper in the snow, before taking off again. To have wings is freedom. Latvia is even smaller than Ireland, but seems large because of its wildness and strange place names like

Ogre. I'll be running to Ogre on the stretch between Riga and Russia.

The magnificent forests almost stretch to the outskirts of the city as if the trees want to march into town to join in the fun. At last on 12 January I make it. I run across a bridge with cannons at the end of it, leading over the Daugava river. It's snowing again and in the midst of it I make out old and new tall spires, a small golden dome on my right and ice fishermen on the river.

I can't believe I'm here. Whatever happens in the future, I've arrived at the first true pitstop of the whole run. It is here that I'm going to have to finalise my visa for Russia and my equipment for the next, formidable stage of my run through Russia and Siberia.

Nothing can take this landmark away.

My father, Major Ronald Ponsonby Griffin, was in Riga as an officer in the British Army long before I was born. I wonder what he would have thought of all this? To be here feels fantastic. I feel like cheering and laughing aloud and shouting out the name *Riga, Riga!*

Too late I realise I'm actually doing so, yelling with joy. People stare, many start yelling and cheering too. It seems that Latvians are like this, full of *joie de vivre*. They must think something incredible is happening, not just me coming in. It makes me run fast, and they shout for me more. Several people throw their hats in the air, catching them neatly, adroitly sticking them back on their heads again before they get too cold.

I run around the city, looking for the main railway station which always seems a good place to find a cheap hotel. Grand gothic buildings give way to the modern city of glitzy shops and nightclubs with windows and doors shaking and leaping to music even at 10am. In dirty, seedy, happy, boisterous streets shops defy gravity by cramming a plethora of bottles of olive oil, sausages, cheeses and everything else on groaning shelves. Being hungry, I immediately find the amazing Rigan black bread the best I've ever tasted. Stalls sell sausages and pancakes; a beggar plays a fiddle with all his heart; people dance to keep warm just as in Lithuania. Pedestrian crossings are never used, I learn at once. To get across the traffic, you attach yourself to a sturdy Rigan woman and face the vehicles down suicidally.

A giant Christmas tree still stands near the station; travellers come and go; sparrows whirl in flocks seeking scraps; seagulls shriek and wheel around the snowy skies; nobody seemed to stay still for here for a moment except patient ice fishermen on the great river.

Situated on the second floor of a tall building, the Aurora Hotel has a heavy wooden door, with dark, dusty stairs leading to it. But the welcome is friendly. My room is small yet six times larger than the bivvi. There are crisply folded white sheets for me to put under the grey blankets. I lie back on the bed, grateful to have made it.

The 1700 miles from Tenby has taken 103 days. Yet the greatest fear and challenge are still ahead: how to be able to run in Russia. There's so much still to do to prepare for that and not a moment to lose, as I have to finalise my Russian visa and get my equipment ready for what may very well be a leap into the unknown.

CHAPTER 12

The Rising of the Phoenix

Latvia, February 2004

My body may still be in Latvia but my mind is running ahead of me.

Russia! The largest country in the world but also so many worlds within worlds. A complex, extraordinary enigma. I feel in some ways I'm jumping over the edge of everything I've known. I don't know how long the 10,000 miles through Russia will take.

Could I really head off through the vast, almost unimaginable landscape of Russia and Siberia? I planned my route two years ago, staring at a map of Siberia, feeling the hair at the back of my neck standing on end, my spine tingling, heart exploding at the thought of going there. Not only has it been the way to go because there's land to run on, but I now realise it's been my passionate goal. I wouldn't have been interested in running around the world in any other way. I'm driven as much by what I don't know as everything I do know.

I've not forgotten Omsk, which I visited during the marathon, and the doctor in the Siberian Railway Hospital who put human guts on a plate during cancer surgery, nor how high the casualties are from cancer, nor everything I learned about the Kitezh Community.

Kitezh means 'The Rising of the Phoenix'. It brings lives back through sheer love and care. Kitezh is a purpose-built village in a forest 300km south of Moscow, where families come to live with their own children and foster children rescued from the streets and impersonal institutions. It was founded by Dimitry Morozov, a Russian despairing at the suffering of orphans in Russia.

Russia is more important to me than ever because I've been in touch with Liza Hollingshead in Britain and Carrie Disney, a dedicated fundraiser for Kitezh, living in Moscow. She's been helping me plan my logistics but also arranging events around my arrival in Moscow, to raise desperately needed funds for Kitezh.

I want to try and help Liza's orphans at the Kitezh Community for Children in Russia. I feel so grateful for my life, to my mother for having me, Marianne and everybody who helped me or brought me up. My grandmother Carlie used to say, 'You're not an orphan if somebody cares about you.' I have always believed dreams can come true. Also that all horizons are narrow – unless I can also in my turn pass on just a little of the bounty I have had.

One child's story, recounted by Liza, illustrates why it matters so much. When Sasha was eight his mother sold him for 10 roubles (about 20p) at a metro station in Moscow. The man who 'bought' him took him to an orphanage where he lived for four years. The rooms had no light, no heat, so he lived in a corridor. He cried bitter tears in every lesson after he'd arrived at Kitezh, because he couldn't answer questions put to children five years younger than himself. He walked alone, couldn't make friends, had nothing to say, thought he had nothing to offer. So they gave him lessons on his own with a loving teacher. His new father took him to work with the bees, taught him how to chop wood; his mother taught him to bake pies. He's beginning to be able to study at school now and make friends. I'm very proud that I am soon to have two Russian goddaughters, Nellie and Marina. Marina's from a family of seven who were rescued. They were so hungry that the youngest, aged only three, tried to eat coal.

Although I'm determined to get to Russia, Riga is one big mother of all pitstops. I have be totally prepared for the next stage. My family, friends and I have always known that the hard part of the run starts here. *Runner's World* are very generously sponsoring me a satphone from Riga onwards, as conditions will become increasingly remote. They will also provide me with a Garmin GPS, which is extremely good of them. Maps, navigation, insurance, visas, documentation, equipment and the practicalities of accessing money from my account in remote places – everything has to be worked out down to the last detail.

Because I have been able to camp most of the time, I have actually spent very little so far – only about £1,000, excluding what I had to pay for foot surgery and kind Nicolas's decadent euros. I am so grateful above all to Ann in Tenby, my fabulous and stoical friend, who is still managing my affairs at home. Ann, a champion runner who finished the Bristol

Half Marathon even when she'd lost a shoe on the way, is as tough as she's golden-hearted. She's always amused me by saying, 'When you're so exhausted that you're nearly unconscious, you've probably still only used up 70% of your energy.' Ann has lived in Tenby for years but comes from Sweden where she was a policewoman. She astounded both criminals and fellow officers, because when she got busy and needed both hands, she put her notebooks down her bra for safekeeping, making one boob twice the size of other. She didn't always use the same side, so nobody ever knew which boob would be the biggest that day.

I spend my first morning in Riga resting and can't stop eating. Next day Geoff arrives like Father Christmas, bringing shoes; the new stove; a fabulous strong replacement bivvi; more down clothing from Peter Hutchinson; thirst-point filter bottles so I can drink even polluted snow-water if I have to; and Kendal Mint Cake from my family. He's told me that yet again he has only had to lift the phone: all the equipment has been given freely. Not even a champion could have better back-up. I am in awe of the kindness I am continually being shown.

I can't get over the fact that Geoff has come out again. It's fantastic to see him and talk about plans. His girlfriend Inna, born in East Siberia, is a brilliant support to me too. Inna lives in London but is away in Moscow visiting her family and has generously accepted the commission from *Runner's World,* amidst a busy life, to pick up the GPS in Moscow so the correct Russian maps can be put on it. This is literally going to save my life as it will get me back on the right track when disaster later strikes in East Siberia.

Without it I'll just become another pile of bones in the forest along with all the other human bones I'll come across.

Mike King comes out to take photos for *Runner's World*, bringing the satphone and solar charger. Geoff also comes out for one day. After he leaves I need to visit Tallinn, Estonia, 200km by bus. I'm not going there on my run, but it's been arranged for me to get my Russian visa there. An essential invitation from St Petersburg, where Liza has friends, has been sent to her contacts in Tallinn and it's hoped the multi-entry visa valid for a year can finally be sorted there. It's complicated: you have to get the visa outside Russia, but you must have the Russian invitation. Even Liza is worried that after all this it might still fail. Tallinn is an exceptionally beautiful city, with conical towers and spires like something out of a Disney movie. Everyone speaks at least five languages. Natalya graciously puts me up and surprisingly the Russian Embassy in Tallinn issue the visa overnight.

Then I have to go to St Petersburg to register my visa. I take the train there feeling slightly anxious: hardly anybody has run alone through Russia and nobody knows what the authorities will really say to such a thing. They took my passport away and kept it for ten days but when it came back, to my relief it was all in order.

St Petersburg is beautiful in the snow, with the Hermitage and Winter Palace and other famous buildings, but it is not a happy place. One night I leave the flat where I've been given accommodation, and there's a dead man outside my door. He's got drunk and has frozen to death.

Nobody takes any notice of him apart from a cat who sits looking at him. He's dressed in rags but is a fine-looking gentleman, reminding me of Topol from *Fiddler on the Roof*. I inform the police, but the following day he's still there. There are homeless people suffering from frostbite in the face, with blood pouring from the blisters, trying to shelter in the subways, drinking just to get oblivious. It's only −20°C, but I've been told this is a killer cold. I wish I could have come back an hour earlier and given him my down jacket if it would have helped him. Somebody loved this man once and his death is such waste. It's also a warning. Life is pitiless and sad here.

While waiting for the visa I work on my writing, have several visits with a dentist who fixes my tooth, and meet Liza's pleasant red-haired friend Inna Yakovleva and her mother, who's survived Hitler's 900-day blockade in 1941/44 during which over a million died from hunger. When even the rats to eat had run out, they boiled glue from their wallpaper to drink.

In retrospect, looking back on the whole of my world run, the irony was that although St Petersburg was not on my route, as I would be running directly east from Riga to Moscow, it had a massive impact on me and was very important in making the rest of my experience in Russia seem clearer.

One bright spot for me is seeing Catherine. She's left Nedd the cat to be spoilt by one of her friends who's specially flown from New York to London for the honour of cat-sitting him. I run to her hotel, dripping melting snow all over the floor as we have breakfast. I am overjoyed to see her. As always she is so thoughtful and caring in every way. She even gives me her luxurious thermal underwear, the only set she has with her. My need is greater, she says.

Finally I'm back in Aurora, ready to run the 970km from Riga to Moscow. So much time has passed but it can't have been otherwise. I get the police to sign my logbook, and finally on Sunday, 8 February, I run out from Riga.

The snow is deep, the going hard. Everything is fine, except the pack is too heavy. On the way to Ogre, my tocs start bleeding, a bad sign. This is because I had very minor frost-bite some months ago, and the skin is more tender.

I fix my eyes on the next snowy tree about 100 yards ahead, sit on the ground and lever the straps of the pack on my back as I can't lift it on, then stagger to my feet and somehow bear the weight on my back until I reach the tree, lean against it to rest, or catch my breath. Then on to the next tree, in a crazy kind of *Fartlek*, or 'interval sessions'. They say in life your aims have to exceed your grasp. I wish this didn't always happen.

I've got used to carrying everything with me for the first 1700 miles, because logistics in sending it ahead would have been very difficult. But now the weight is very much greater and I'm going to have to do something about it.

Clive would have smiled. He always thought vets knew best and my mind goes back to Martin, the Marlborough vet, and his advice about getting a buggy to pull instead of carry-ing a backpack. I decide I'll definitely get a cart or pushchair, though that might have to wait until Moscow.

I have to cope but I can lessen the load. The most critical problem is that the satphone has a heavy solar panel which is difficult to lash safely onto the backpack. It's also vital that I don't damage the solar panel as it will be essential for me in the wilderness.

I find out from the manager of Ogre service station that I should be able to get a cheap mobile phone for the immediate area – but not yet. Fortunately I've made contact with Colonel Grant, UK Defence Attaché in Riga, who also happens to be a distinguished pentathlete who ran for Great Britain. We hadn't met in Riga but have spoken on the phone. I call him from Ogre. He instantly grasps the problem and sends his driver out to collect the phone, solar panel, heavy camera and other things into his safekeeping to be dispatched in the diplomatic bag to the embassy in Moscow. I call Steven Seaton to explain what I'm doing and he's going to order me a smaller electrical charger to supplement the solar panel when possible.

After that I get on much better. The new bivvi and stove are excellent. Although the snow is deeper and the weather worse than before Riga, everything feels so much easier as the new bivvi has an extra strong zip. It's bliss to be able to shut out the storms and cook again. Heaven to make simple hot meals and drinks along the road and melt snow again even for a little makeshift hot-water bottle again at night. The down clothes and bags also keep me warm. As the temperature plunges for a brief spell to –30°C at night, it seems like magic.

From Ogre I carry on along little roads parallel to the Daugava River and highway, avoiding lorries spewing black smoke into white-outs. The small places on the roads are so friendly that struggling through often deep snow to use them is well worthwhile. In a tiny place called Krape, Mr Gatis, a teacher, lets me use his computer to email James for the first time since Riga. I love the idea that his website is making friends I may never meet but who are thinking of me and will be part of my life for ever.

In Plavinas, where I arrive on 13 February, I post letters and call home, getting news of Eve and the others like my sister Maude, and Marianne who's trying to send me a tiny bottle of Fabergé perfume, which will weigh nothing, she says, and will bring memories of good times and elegance back to me when things are at their hardest to keep me going. She's sending it via Carrie Disney in Moscow.

This is beginning to feel like a personal place to me.

CHAPTER 13

To Russia with Love

Latvia–Russia, February 2004

Over the next ten days I plod and trot on through Varajklani, bypassing Rezekne and camp near the village of Tutani. The snow is deep in the woods and it snows even more at night. I'm quite worried about being able to get out of it.

Eating is always the answer. I make spaghetti though I pour half of it away by accident while emptying the water out. Hungrily, I scoop it back into the pan again, snow and all, and eat it chilled and tasty. Delia Smith and the Naked Chef couldn't have done a better job.

There's a little fuel station further on in the next small place, the attendant locked in like a prisoner for the sake of security. No food to buy, no payphone. I miss the sat and must get a phone soon. Next morning I arrive at the friendly town of Ludsa, with gleaming frozen lakes reflecting pink in a rare, sublime winter sunset. I stay in a little hotel for two nights while the doctor looks at my sore feet, giving them laser treatment which he's certain is the answer.

I'm now within 54km of the Russian border.

* * *

A lady rushes out from a wooden farmhouse in the middle of the forest asking me in, as it's snowing heavily. They're nice and hospitable but have drunk a lot of vodka and speak a strange dialect of Latvian. The lady, Katya, says I must be tired (according to my phrasebook) and shows me this lovely big bed. I thank her and at once fall fast asleep.

When I wake up there are six people in the bed. The wife is next to me and her husband is on the other side of her. He seems to be having bad dreams and hitting her affectionately in his sleep, but hits me as well as his arms are so long. A drunken son is at the bottom of the bed; another man and several children are sleeping around the edges.

A boiler, which has fired itself up during the night, makes the room scorching. Sweat is pouring from everyone, including me. When they get up, I don't let them know I'm surprised as it might hurt their feelings.

Katya keeps opening drawers in the ramshackle kitchen, determined to make sandwiches for me. All the drawers she opens, sighing and shrugging in disappointment, are filled with vodka bottles until she gets to the last one where she finds the bread. She lifts it out and a mouse jumps out at the same time, but she makes the sandwiches just fine.

I'm left with a lingering impression of how nice they are, and hope life is going OK for them.

I'm fourteen days from Riga, including two and a half rest days. On the evening of 22 February I'm within sight of the Russian border. My heart is jumping all over the place. There's no point in fooling myself that the easy trip to St

Petersburg to get the visa means I will actually make it on foot. I think back when I was in London before I set out. The agencies told me I could be put in jail if I tried to get in with a business visa. Nobody, not even Liza Hollingshead, is sure what will happen when I actually reach the border alone and on foot. The time has come to find out.

I approach Russia at night. I hesitate, just like I did when I was approaching Lithuania. The only time I fear the dark is when I am approaching the border of a new country. It is never the best time to deal with uncertainties. I stand still and gaze ahead. It looks peaceful. The lights of the lorries waiting to cross the border are stopped like a city on wheels. Steam rises from the drivers' mugs of tea as they get out of their cabs for a stretch or a pee, and hang out with their friends. Vodka is being handed around to keep warm and there's a busy makeshift kiosk selling food. They look at me curiously as I arrive. The situation seems at once volatile and peaceful. A great tit, probably from Russia, hops around my feet, saying hello.

I'm very anxious and decide to cross the border in the morning. I walk back into the forests, making the bivvi snug among the beautiful pine trees. Out of sight from the lights of the lorries, it becomes the darkest of nights. Not a star in the sky, not a breath of wind. I'm alone with my thoughts. *Shall I get across the border? Will I have trouble after all?*

I'm haunted by the warnings. Peter Smith, British Consul General in Moscow, wrote to me concerned. He is worried I'll run out of food, get pushed off the road by drunken drivers, be hurt or get in trouble. He fears I might be lost and lie for days without being found. He's risen magnificently to the occasion after being assured I'm well equipped and prepared, and he is apparently producing an extraordinary letter or document, like the old-fashioned travellers' passport Dame Freya Stark carried in the early twentieth century along the lines of 'I was a good and faithful subject of Great Britain, and to help me'; but the warnings from such a source have to be taken seriously.

Dawn breaks. I pass along the lines of lorries, whose drivers give me tea. I approach the Customs Post; they take my passport, look at it carefully and start talking to each other while I wait. There about five officers, including two women in green uniforms with orange lapels and two in different uniforms who seem to be policemen.

They all look so serious. Suddenly they begin smiling and say, '*Ohsin priatna, Aileen, Rosita.*' Aileen's my first Christian name in my passport. I've been trying to learn more Russian and know this is a friendly greeting. It means something like 'You are welcome here'. They just wave me on my way.

I'm in such a hurry to get going, having received their blessing and before they change their minds, that I slip and fall on the icy road, whereupon one of the police picks me up like a puppy, putting me back on my feet. The other policeman comes up, opening his purse. I think this is one of the fines I must pay that I've been told about, but no: according to an officer who speaks a little English, apparently he just wants to give me 50 roubles because his mother has a cafe in the next village where she makes special soups, and he wants to treat me.

*   *   *

I wander along the road thinking how strange it is to be in Russia. It's been too easy and I'm still uncertain. It's getting dark again. I run until about 4 pm. I'm in a different time-zone, one hour ahead from yesterday.

When I pass the border, I mention something about staying with friends, but of course that would be 600km ahead in Moscow. I'm not sure if they'd understand about the camping. So I go down the first small side road; it's snowing heavily again which covers my footsteps. I plunge into the forest, curling up in the bivvi in all my warm bags. I don't light my stove or use my torch, just stay very quietly. I'm not sure what would happen if someone found me, if it would be OK or not. But nothing happens and next morning I'm back on the road.

Suddenly the policemen are there again. If I've broken the law this would be very serious for me: they have the power and right to stop me camping. But unless I do so, I can't continue the journey because the distances all through Russia are too great. This is a pivotal moment. I start trying to explain then suddenly see a change in their expressions. They don't care at all. They laugh and say they like having a tourist here. One officer seizes me in a bear-hug, swinging me round and round before setting me back down on my feet carefully.

The bear-hug is surprising; but it seems to mean that everything is all right. I later learn that a hug is a mark of respect in Russia. If you only like someone a bit, you shake their hands or simply embrace cordially. But to be swung around, that's a real honour.

*   *   *

By Wednesday, 25 February, I'm within 50km of Pustoshka. I've been to the tiny cafe in the forest, owned by the officer's mother. It is dwarfed by gigantic lorries parked all around in a muddy forest clearing. The only place to eat in a hundred miles, they say. The soup is robust: the spoon almost stands up by itself. Later, when I have to eat spaghetti with reindeer hairs and lumps of grit in it, I dream of this soup. The lady at the cafe also changes my Latvian roubles into Russian roubles.

I keep thinking how beautiful Russia is: deep green firs with clumps of snow on them and icicles hanging from the ends of the branches like chandeliers. The first part of the M9 in Russia isn't like motorways anywhere else: it's fairly empty in the 100km between the Latvian border and Velikie Luci. Occasional overladen HGV lorries rush along the road, but hardly a car. Giving the lorry drivers a wave makes them toot or flash their lights at me. This cheers me along the way because loneliness is an enemy. There's only so much you can say to yourself. The weight of the pack is considerable and starts to make my back go into spasms and cramps; my hips are clicking and hurting. The pain is a distraction to the loneliness but it is still an unwelcome one.

It's fantastic arriving at Velikie Luki three days later and having a bath. Here I find the first ATM machine since long before the Latvian border, and obtain more roubles, as I've begun to get very low and have been eking them out. Many people along this stretch of highway in Russia say there's nothing along the edge of the road. You'll find nothing for days but on foot you see shanty places and tiny shops. They've kept me going.

As for the hotel in Velikie Luki, it may not be the Hilton, it isn't like the one in Leer either or the Aurora, but it's a seven-star hotel to me. The dark, damp corridors actually lead to a room with its own bath. And though the water looks rusty orange, this doesn't bother me at all. I use up a whole bottle of cheap shampoo I've bought to wash myself and the clothes. I also take apart the Omni multi-fuel stove. It can burn almost anything but objects to Russian petrol and smokes black clouds of soot every time. I clean it, carefully bagging all the sooty particles to avoid making a mess. Then, as steam from my clothes drying on the radiators fills the room, I bask in the resulting sauna and fall fast asleep.

CHAPTER 14

Unstoppable Friend

Russia, February–March 2004

Much more shameful than being frightened is being frightening. Like the experts say, Russia isn't a clear place to take in. My discoveries tear my heart.

During the first 150km I haven't as yet encountered road rage or drunken driving. As for theft, when I drop my purse by accident in Pustoshka, a tall man on a bicycle, with a child perched on in front, comes after me and hands it back. It's honesty but somehow more than that – pride, a mask saying, 'I'm Russian, I'm doing OK.' Never before my time in Russia have I experienced such fierce determination to disguise pain and need. I tie some money in a bag to the collar of their small dog while petting it, as they won't take a reward, even though they look badly dressed for the weather. My life will never be so dangerous and hard as for the people I've already met in the countryside; people nearly hidden, like the shanties and shops I've only discovered on foot. Blink twice and you'd miss them.

I approach some tiny houses a day after leaving Velikie Luki. I have a problem as the snow is seven foot deep at the side of the road. I can't get into it to put the bivvi up as I'm becoming submerged. There are some desperately poor-looking wooden and tin shacks with what looks like a rick of straw beneath mounds of snow beside a tumbledown building or shed. The door opens and a woman comes out in heavy headscarf and big boots, holding a pail.

She stares when she sees me approach. I stop but she cries out, dropping the pail. Milk runs all over the snow. I knock on her door as I'm so sorry and want to recompense for the milk. The door stays shut, so does the next door. Then faces and movement appear at the windows and a sharp voice shouts out to a child to hurry in, as far as I can understand.

At the very last house a light comes on because it's getting dark, and a couple come out. They're waving and calling to me. I have enough Russian to explain what I'm doing and say I'm sorry. They shrug their shoulders and smile. The wife puts her arms around me. They make tea and find berries for me to try, which she says they gather in the forest in the summer. Then the lady I frightened comes in at last. They show me the cow. It's white with beautiful big brown eyes. She has a warm blanket on her back to keep her cosy, they say, so she'll give more milk.

The lady starts talking in English that I hadn't realised she understood, and says they bought the cow cheaply from the slaughterhouse, because she had a cracked foreleg and limped, but she gives milk just fine and that's why she's been saved. They couldn't have afforded a cow otherwise. I don't stay, because I feel I can manage now. It's all in the head.

* * *

They say silver birches called *birosova* and spruce trees in Russia protect each other. When pine trees are tall and mighty, the young silver birches grow in their shelter. Then, when the birches are tall, they stand guard over the next crop of little spruces. That's why they naturally grow and are found in these forests together in a kind of cycle. Trees are inspiring and comforting. The pieces of fir tree branch and twigs on the ground also make excellent makeshift snow shoes.

I tie the bivvi out straight so it can't sink, as the snow is so soft. It's become much milder tonight. I make the mistake of climbing into it too slowly and a torrent of watery snow pours in with me, but the old system holds good. The bags are wet but my inner layers are waterproof. I sleep immediately and don't even have any dreams.

I wake early, stick my head out like a fox, climb out and have a good shake. The landscape is a fairytale-looking white. It looks as if winter will last forever, but suddenly I hear it, almost a whisper: a new soft swishing or gentle crackling. I see the gleam on the snow. It glimmers. There's nothing dramatic, it's just starting to melt. I can hear action in the trees that have been empty and silent.

The tree near me has become alive with little birds. They're not only chirping or making the lonely sounds. They've begun busily twittering as if in a kind of a fuss, and full of it. Then I hear a blackbird sing for the first time in Russia. I lie there in awe. The winter is being beaten.

I can't see spring around the corner yet but I can hear it. Lying out there in the snow by myself this morning I can hardly describe my feelings. I've been unaware how on a run alone, it's little things like this that can squeeze your heart with both joy and pain. I feel weak but also strengthened by memories of love and sweetness. That's what the song of a blackbird always does.

2 March – a beautiful day. I'm excited because Carrie Disney, who is my link with Kitezh, is going to drive out from Moscow to hunt me down. It will be great to meet her. In her emails to Eve, James, Geoff and others she's amused me by referring to me as 'our unstoppable friend', but it's Carrie who's really the unstoppable one. She's the very first to come out and meet me on the road in Russia. I pass the 461km marker when a large car draws up and Carrie jumps out. She later writes:

> It was a beautiful morning – cold and clear with milky light, and the road was long and straight – quite a few heavy lorries, but not much other traffic. I had spotted a few road signs in the distance, and been convinced they were Rosie; then we saw a moving road sign in the distance, and it was Rosie. You really couldn't tell whether she was a man or a woman, as there wasn't more than half an inch of skin exposed to the elements. She had hat and face mask, and gloves and scarves and three layers of trousers, and still managed a cheery wave as we slowed to stop in front of her.

Carrie has a merry face, and wild fair hair sticking out from under her big hat. She's closely followed by an enchanting-looking shaggy lurcher dog. A slim man with steady green eyes and charming smile also gets out of the car. She introduces

him as Sasha, the personal driver of her partner Richard Tickner, chief executive at Moscow's HSBC bank. Sasha, a real star,
has been 'lent' for the day, giving up his time, because Carrie
doesn't yet have a Russian driving licence.

They've come because Carrie has a fabulous letter for me
from Peter Smith, British Consul General in Moscow. Carrie
emphasises that Sir Roderic and Lady Lyne, British Ambassador and his wife, have been the power in the background
for the tremendous support. Carrie has other things for me
and is anxious to feed me a good breakfast, especially because
the temperature in the last hours has dropped from freezing
to –11°C again, and is forecast to be –17 by night-time.

There's nowhere around here so we plan that I'll stop at
the 461km mark and set off from here again later and drive
back to Velikie Luki, not so far by car. It's fun. Dora the
lurcher has decided to become my lapdog, which is quite a
honour. She's gorgeous. Carrie tells me that gypsies' lurchers
are very opinionated· they have to persuade themselves they
like you before they'll even sit on your lap as a blanket

At the little hotel they welcome me as if I'm coming home.
One lady jokes that if I'd run around the world already, I
must have gone pretty fast. I don't stop talking or eating for
at least an hour. I realise it's the first time since Riga that I've
been able to talk English freely, and I can't stop myself. As
Carrie later writes in an email for the website:

> I don't think she drew breath for about half an hour. She
> had so much to tell us. I suspected that she was starved in
> another sense, as she polished off seven large buns and four
> cups of coffee.

They're horrified to learn my sleeping bags are soaking wet. Sasha whisks them back to the car where he turns the engine on and cleverly dries the sleeping bags by placing them between the engine and bonnet. I wouldn't have allowed anyone else to do this. The bags are my lifeline, but there's something about Sasha I profoundly trust. It works too. By the time we leave, the bags are all dry so I have a lovely bed tonight.

When Carrie joined Richard out in Moscow, she became, as she put it, 'a trailing spouse'. She wants to use her time to make a difference. She's devastated by orphanages in Russia where children are left in their cots alone for so many hours they get flat heads and where infants sometimes have their bottoms washed under the tap in icy water their carers don't bother to heat. It's taken her over completely when, after much research, she's discovered Kitezh.

What a force Kitezh is for the good. Out of the original desperate streetkids and those from grim institutions that it has saved, four have won university places, and all have gone on to lead useful, happy lives, thanks to patience, loving care and attention. The planning for events she's arranging, including a run I'm to do with the Kitezh children around Moscow to Red Square, a reception at the British Embassy and other venues, is going from strength to strength.

Finally we return to the 461km mark. They've had to get up at 5am so it's decided that Sasha will drive ahead and have a sleep, while Carrie and I walk together, with Dora bouncy and enthusiastic on a long lead.

10km later, we say goodbye – and I carry on alone.

CHAPTER 15

Paw-prints in the Snow

Russia, March 2004

Purpose is everything. Yet the purpose is harder to achieve than the running itself. It has both shattered and strengthened me that I can sleep outside in the snow at −20°C, even manage without hot food, curl up like a stray puppy on the side of the road, yet I can shout at the wind and nobody's listening.

The run was conceived through circumstances that tore me apart and will be no good unless it's of some use. The greatest wonder and joy have been how Eve and James picked the purpose up and held it to them. Eve has painstakingly typed the scant messages I have often just spoken from some callbox and James has somehow kept the website going. Thousands are now following the run, which means everything as there have been letters from people who have said their lives have been saved because they have been for health checks. Meeting Carrie has made me hope to help the Kitezh orphans more too.

I can hardly wait for Moscow. I'm sensing that the reasons for running are growing in all kinds of ways, some unspoken. I know now that the run is for everyone: for the girls with scarlet and green hair in Lithuania; the lady with her white cow, whom I had frightened; the truckers hooting me; the man with no legs; and the little girl who rushed out to give me sweets on the very first day in Wales. Also for those I can't meet. The run is my responsibility but it's not mine alone; it belongs to people who've touched it and will touch it. This is going to become more important than could be imagined.

It's soon only 300km to the capital, at the moment I run 17 to 20 km a day. The nights are still long and there is a spell-bindingly surreal light in the woods. The moon has caught the branches of the silver birches, making it look as if the trees are shining.

I've gone deeper into the forest than usual to find a dry little place among the melting snow. It seems very peaceful. Suddenly a loud crashing in the trees tears the forest apart. I sit up shaking and hit my head on the bivvi canvas that's not tall enough for this. Little icicles from the condensation fly down my neck and calm me down. Then I don't hear anything else.

It goes silent, except for the hooting of an owl. I've always thought of the forest as my protector, the darkness too. I haven't been afraid of the dark since childhood. I used to have to herd the cows for milking at 5am. In winter the lantern would go out and I'd sometimes fall over a sleeping cow. This crash sounds enormous, but sounds can be illusions and the forest has its own voices. You never know.

I keep listening and looking out. There's nothing to see but the moonlight with a rainbow ring around the moon's edge flooding the forest floor in all its grandeur. At last I can't help falling asleep again, I'm so tired.

I look out next morning. There are giant clawmarks in the snow. These are bear pawprints coming right up to where I've been sleeping. They go all around the bivvi. I stare at them, stunned and shaking. I can't get over that a bear has woken up from his hibernation and come over to visit. And I've never known anything about it at all.

Then I hear the sound of the first running stream of the year close by. I've read that when bears first wake up they search for fresh clean water as they're always dehydrated and thirsty before even being hungry after their long sleep.

It's dangerous to run from a bear. I knew that wildlife would be part of my journey as it's always been and that it would be getting larger. I knew I'd have to cope; the secret must be there on how to do it, but not this morning. Just now I don't think I'll ever be able to look at fresh large pawprints in the snow and not feel shaky.

He doesn't come back. I pack up and head off quietly.

Over the next few days catkins are coming out on the bushes so fast they seem to be growing as I look; and the thunder of ice cracking apart beneath the snow makes me leap with fright. The snow is still deep. I try to imagine Russia without snow. Arriving in a country under snow is almost parallel to getting to somewhere at night, wondering what will unfold when you can see the land. Except that the snow with all its shapes and illusions is more potent and mysterious than the darkness can ever be. It doesn't hide land; it creates ideas of its own and takes you and sways you.

Now the birds are in pairs, sitting on bare branches; they and the plants far beneath the snow know their time is coming. Spring is more than sounds now; it's becoming visible. Spring is on the brink.

My fuel bottle has started leaking petrol. I'm without the use of my stove again and my hip is a bit sore but I know the hip and bottle only have to wait to be fixed up in Moscow. It's very difficult to carry enough food in the backpack as distances are quite long. I can't wait to get a cart to pull. Sometimes I'm full up, and sometimes very hungry. A great salvation is oat flakes and hunks of fat called *sala*, so solid that it has a lot of calories; a chunk of *sala* is a great emergency larder.

Russia is like Brigadoon. Some little villages you see on the map don't exist when you get there. Others appear out of nowhere. I've just passed a sign saying in the Russian alphabet (which I can now decipher) 'Cafe 80km'. I find it about a hundred yards away. It's just a box, tilted on its side with icicles from the roof to the ground and steam coming out of a little chimney. It's occupied, and it's a hotel too. There are several boxes scattered among the trees and the welcome is tremendous. As for the cooking, thick stew and *gresca*, or buckwheat – it's sensational. The box with a bed in it only costs the equivalent of three US dollars. Best of all is the barman. He even makes a brew of old tins which he melts down in the tiny garage next to the boxes and pours into my fuel bottle, making a kind of weld so I can use my stove again.

On 12 March I arrive in the pristine Volga valley, still frozen by winter. Boats are laid up but the fishermen are at their ice-holes. It has the air of a frontier town, with trucks and drivers and their mechanics, instead of horses and cowboys; a partly hidden town off the main highway, now much busier and fiercer with extra lanes. I see several black limousines parked among the lorries. There's a babble of voices as doors open and men in smart suits, some wearing gold Rolexes, pile out. They're probably just here for the Russian elections taking place in two days. They are polite and curious. I find *peshcom* and *bijam*, meaning walking or running, two very useful Russian words, and head off to a little store selling aspirin for my hip.

14 March is Election Day – Putin has been re-elected. There's 20% more traffic on the highway and things get even busier before Moscow. The police stop and ask for my papers, and I'm allowed to carry on in style.

A gleaming stretch limousine draws up next. Three burly men get out and try to tell me I can't be on foot here. Then a slim man, short but standing tall, emerges. He has silvery hair and eastern features, a nice face. He listens and says he's from Yakutia in Siberia; and bows and shakes my hand. 'Travel with your heart, not with your feet,' he says in perfect English, apparently telling the men to back off. I'll never know what all this is about.

'You're the first person I've ever met from Siberia,' I tell him, feeling pleased. Then they're off as mysteriously as they arrived.

My hip is still hurting, my toes are bleeding a little as I bumped them on some sharp ice a few days ago in the woods, but the discomfort is worth it as it is so exciting to get past Volokolamsk. I have been travelling on the M9 but it becomes an expressway closer to the MKAD, the great big ring road around Moscow, so I dodge on and off the smaller roads. There's forest for wide stretches, and deep snow; it's partly melting and the ice refreezes as the weather gets warmer, then becomes cold again. I'm reminded that this is Russia and it's only the second week of March. With all the hustle and bustle of the traffic, this forest where I'm still camping most nights is now like the veneer, just as the road seemed to be before.

The change is more profound than that. After all the loneliness and isolation, time is a kaleidoscope: so much happens. I suddenly get more kind attention on the ground than I've ever had before. I wonder if it would have been better if all the journey had been like this: PR and more chance of raising sponsorship.

Dena, a young Kitezh volunteer, arrives with Jennifer, a physio generously offering her treatment free to me. They bring food, a phone and news; and Jennifer treats my hip in a village cafe, while her husband Pavel and two-year-old son distract the amazed waitress. They confirm the original plan. A fundraising launch at Carrie's home on 20 March is extremely critical: the British Ambassador is going to be there. Sasha will pick me up on the 19th from wherever I've reached and we'll make a note of the km marker. He'll put me back afterwards because my aim is to run to Red Square.

The *Moscow Times* come out and the journalist is a lady originally from Wales called Rebecca, another first on this run. Several Russian TV stations send cameramen and presenters. The cars are often unmarked but you know what they are before you even see the camera because first out is the reporter who's nearly always a glamorous woman teetering in high heels on the ice, yet moving faster than I can. The only other interviews until now were the one with the Polish newspapers where I didn't understand the questions or answers. But this time they all speak English or have translators for what I say.

Next, thanks to James, BBC World TV pick up the story. Sara Rainsford and Zoya, the directors, and Valli Kaub, the cameraman, come and make a film that will be seen by 200 million people worldwide. I hope it does some good for the charity as they don't believe in half measures. Award-winning Valli nearly seems to kill himself as he lies on his stomach on the ice, filming my feet. They follow me into the forest, immortalising the little stove. It isn't grateful at all: it's smoking on the low-grade Russian petrol, and also because the night has got colder I keep having to relight it. So I have a black sooty face, as I can tell by the expressions of the film crew, as well as icicles for earrings. It's amazing how when you don't have a mirror the best way to tell how you look is from the amused glances on other people's faces.

The phone is very useful to make a rendezvous. '*Kak dila* – how are you?' Sasha greets me. He speaks beautiful English, but I'm trying to learn Russian. Sasha eventually collects me from the road near a little place called Krasnogorsk just 45km from Red Square.

I sit there, watching the buildings fly past as if on fast-forward after all this time on foot, past the markets, the suburbs, cafes and tall banks and glittering buildings, past signs for the metro and the bright lights that weren't there when I last saw Moscow when I came on a brief visit at the age of eighteen. It seems so quick but I'm seeing the course. This is the first time I've ever had the back-up to go ahead of myself.

The plan is that after this reception I'll go back and run through here. We arrive at last at the little lane called Romanov Pereulok, bang in the centre near Red Square and the Kremlin. Carrie and Richard live on the sixth floor of a large building here.

'Hello, unstoppable friend,' she says, giving me a hug.

It's so great to stop and relax. Richard is tall, courteous, softly spoken. Dora the lurcher seems pleased to see me and I also meet Puff, a fluffy marmalade cat, and Dragon, a sleek, black one.

A short while later I'm sitting in a luxurious bath drinking a glass of white wine and somehow managing to eat a slice of cake at the same time. It's my first bath for six months. A real celebration. I'm being so spoilt and cared for. Memories of icicles breaking off taps, or washing in freezing showers or melted snow, disappear immediately.

After that I'm ready for a party. The reception on 20 March goes well. I could write about the eloquent speeches, the cream of the glittering Russian and English society in Moscow, the Ambassador and his wife Mandy, and all the journalists; being asked to talk about my run and its reasons as I mingle in a blue borrowed skirt. Best of all is meeting Masha, Vasily, Sergey and the Kitezh founder, Dimitry.

Vasily, once facing a hopeless future at a grim orphanage, came to live at the Kitezh village deep in the forest. Loved and educated, he is now about to study law at university.

Sergey, who with his brother ran away from drunken parents when they were six and eight, lived on the streets in the course of which they ran away from five or six orphanages. He's now a talented carpenter with a love of literature, and a twinkle in his eye.

Masha is the natural daughter of Tamara, one of the foster parents. Not only the parents but the children share everything with those taken in.

My next job is to complete my run to Red Square, then make a trip to the Kitezh village deep in the forest near Kaluga, to keep my promises.

CHAPTER 16

Kitezh: Bad Times Can End

Russia, March–April 2004

Two little girls aged about eight run towards me, taking hold of my hands as if they'd never let go. I don't choose my Russian goddaughters; they choose me. Nellie has dancing brown eyes, curling dark hair; Marina bluey green eyes with long fair hair all down her back. They hardly leave my side during my two days there. Nothing I've read or heard about Kitezh prepares me for what I find. There are about 35 children living at the village when I visit: teenagers going down to the youngest, four-year-old twins, and many caring adults.

I'm looking at the children's faces shining with health and exuberance; with restrained giggles, politely prepared welcome and huge sense of fun; and think about the well of suffering in their past lives; the beatings, starvation, being abandoned or cooped up in orphanages that were grey institutions. I remember what I learned about Russian pride and know passionately and almost with anger that Kitezh doesn't deserve help out of pity because of where the children came from, but because of where they're going to and all they've risen above. And I know that nobody will ever be able to do more for the children than these children would do for themselves. Bad times *can* end. Anyone can achieve almost anything, with love.

My new friends sweep me off to show me around. A beautiful lime and birch tree forest and the glimpse of a bright lake beyond are the backdrop for the church, ten or eleven log cabins, and a building I'm to learn is the Playhouse, where children who've never had toys before are taught to play and get over their fears. Little wooden walkways lie between the cabins over the forest clearing and the now rather soggy spring ground. There's a vegetable garden and tiny farm with two cows to give milk for the children, and other animals including a friendly little dog and a ginger kitten found on the Moscow Metro.

'If you give children a beautiful place to live, and with care and education, some of the outer beauty spreads to the inside,' says Dimitry Morozov, founder of Kitezh, with something more than emotion in his face.

I know Kitezh's story well. That's why I decided to run for them back in the UK. Dimitry had to make a stand. Fostering was an unknown concept in Russia. Children put into orphanages stayed there, forgotten, out of sight; hope, life and expectations given to them were so meagre that, when they were eventually released, many ended up on the streets, and 30% died often from suicide and despair within three years.

Kitezh was founded in 1992. Dimitry and his friends decided they wouldn't rest until Russian orphanages were replaced by child-centred family communities; that the only natural way for children is to be part of a family; and to make even the smallest start with this was very important. They'd been given 100 hectares of unwanted land in the forest. He left his job as a radio journalist and he and his friends, many like him with their own young families, set out to do something to educate orphan children and give them love and a sense of belonging within a family.

So Kitezh began with one small house, an outside toilet and a well, the only source of water. They survived like this even in winter with howling winds and temperatures of −20. Four of the original streetchildren they rescued have gone to university, and all have gone on to lead happy, fulfilled lives. It's all grown from there. The village has gained international recognition for therapeutic education and a hundred children have benefited. As the older ones graduate, others are taken in, but life there is still very hard.

I'm very moved by the story of one boy who wouldn't stay at Kitezh unless all his brothers and sisters still stuck in an orphanage could come too. So they did, but it had been difficult: money and space are still short. The kitchens in the small cabins double up as shower room, with the showerhead coiled behind the kitchen sink. Many of the classrooms where the students catch up with years of lost education are bedrooms by night. And the big communal main kitchen and dining hall in the evening becomes a theatre, where the children put on shows.

Against all odds, students have managed to stage a production of *Jesus Christ Superstar* that has toured Moscow and gained awards among school theatres. They put on a wonderful show while I'm there. A funny skit, 'Sad Cow', has me rolling about; Nellie, Marina and others are all dressed up in another sketch and win first prize. Fourteen-year-old Valya plays Mary Magdalen in fabulous scenes from *Jesus Christ Superstar*.

Valya comes up to me afterwards and says, 'Next time you come to Kitezh, I'll teach you how to dance.' I'll definitely take her up on it.

Nellie and Marina, with shining eyes, lead the way to Tamara's cabin to share their prize with me: a box of chocolates, a rare treat as their diet is wholesome and nutritious but doesn't include many fancy delicacies.

All the teachers and carers have foster children, but Tamara is the one I get to know best. She epitomises Kitezh. Tamara Pichugina and her own daughters Nellie and Masha came to Kitezh in spring 2000. She also has eight foster children, including Marina, sister to the boy Volodya who won't stay in Kitezh without his siblings. He's worried about his family and keeps saying, 'If you want to help, do it now.'

Tamara, who also runs the nursery school, says, 'I've found my purpose in life. I love children. Of course it's many clothes to wash, but it's worth it to see the need for love shining from their eyes.'

Nellie and Marina decide to be my god-daughters and it could hardly mean more to me; Nellie bubbling and outgoing, happy to share everything with her new brothers and sisters; and Marina formerly too shy to say a word, I'd been told, and malnourished and thin, but now so full of fun. There shouldn't be divisions on this earth between people; between children who are orphans and others.

One of the greatest gifts Tamara gives me is her lessons about Russian diet; especially *gresca*, or buckwheat, which is of huge value on my journey. Buckwheat is called 'food for warriors' in Russia. Tamara tells me a vitamin in the buckwheat is especially good for helping the circulation during cold weather.

I have to say goodbye to Kitezh, but I'll be back. Dear sweet Nellie and Marina, you haven't made a good choice in me as I'm on the road and shan't be able to send you presents for ages or see you, but you are the symbols of Kitezh for me and I shall always remember you.

A bunch of children come to Moscow with me in the Kitezh minibus and stay with Carrie and Richard. They all do hurdles over the sofas including Dora the lurcher. The next day we take part in a Fun Run arranged by the Hash House Harriers of Moscow, taking in Red Square, St Basil's, the walls of the Kremlin and the banks of the Moskva River. I have the easy part as Dora is with me on a lead, pulling me along, and we end up at the British Ambassador's residence.

A few more days of fundraising after the children have gone home pass in a blur. During the reception itself, hosted by Sir Rodric (a dedicated marathon runner) and Lady Lyne, the little tent was put up in a grand room. The children were absolute stars and several more thousands of dollars were raised. Carrie wrote, 'These funds are incomings during the week/ten days you were in Moscow. Much more was raised indirectly. The fact that you helped me raise the profile of Kitezh meant that we were able to get funding from various organisations to help. The second Kitezh village called Orion was started and is well under way.'

That's so important to me. Every time I look up at my favourite stars in the wilderness skies over the next 10,000 miles, I think of those children and hope I've done something to help them.

It's typical of Carrie that she has not forgotten to arrange a full medical check-up for me at the SOS Clinic in Moscow or help me obtain a visa for Kazakhstan, which I'll have to pass through on my way to Siberia; and has also fixed for DHL to sponsor me and send equipment ahead into the wilds, even to places whose names I can't read or recognise on the map but which will make all the difference.

On 2 April I finally leave Moscow, setting off from Red Square. I'm waved away by Liza and Carrie and a crowd of friends, continuing my track eastwards. I'm 100km from Moscow when a car draws up and Lynne, a friend of Carrie's, jumps out, beaming from ear to ear with excitement. She has a present for me, she announces.

She gets it out as if she were Santa Claus, producing a baby-jogger from Mothercare in Moscow that I shall call Columbine after the old horse I loved when I was a child. The backpack fits in it perfectly. What a joy and relief. I've looked around some of the markets in Moscow, but haven't seen anything suitable. I've forgotten how hard it is with a backpack.

Columbine has instructions saying it's an 'urban jogger' and can take 'slightly uneven pavements'. It ends up going over the Ural Mountains but there are to be many adventures on the way.

CHAPTER 17

The Axeman Cometh

Russia, April–May 2004

One of the men is hitting my hands with the butt of his knife and laughs. I yell with pain and rage but don't let go the handles of the pushchair but these two thickset men who've jumped out at me from the forest about 500km east of Moscow also have hold of it. They have the most vicious faces I've ever seen and make me shiver, the kind of people who pick the wings off flies and then laugh about it. And they're trying to drag me into the forest …

'Come with us,' they say. 'Just for a while.'

'That's not the best way to persuade me.' The butt of the knife is hard and the blade that's pointing away from me is shimmering and sharp. It's as if they think they're strong enough to force me into the woods without the knife. If I let them take me, I think, I may never come back. I'm alone and they are cowards.

It's a beautiful morning. Sunshine streams through the birches' green fresh leaves, making dappled patterns on the road's edge. The birds are singing, the wind is whispering. All this goes through my mind in a fleeting instant: what a strange setting for danger. I look around and, like a hunted animal, see that I must do something that goes completely against my nature.

A gigantic double-trailer truck, maybe on its way to the Urals, is heading along the road between the endless trees, like a great ship in a shipping channel, rushing headlong towards us. I can't wrest away the men's grip, but somehow I turn the nose of Columbine straight into the path of the oncoming lorry. It speeds up, as if maybe the driver wants to avoid trouble, then swerves wildly to avoid running me down. Fumes and grit fly and it misses me by inches. My attackers are surprised enough to let go for a moment. Then I *run*. And run and run … and still have my pushchair. I don't hear the men's footsteps.

I know I mustn't look back. If they're still there, looking back will encourage them, but eventually I bend down quickly as if to check my shoelaces, so I can see backwards. The road is clear and empty. Then I see them way back among the trees, still following me, trying, it seems, to stay hidden. The only good thing is that one has on a bright red shirt and the other a yellow one, so I can spot them.

I run for hours. Suddenly, I can't manage to go any further. I'm exhausted. I still have my equipment, that's the trump card. Columbine is hanging in. The road gets more twisted. I turn a sharp corner and they're out of sight for a moment. I rush into the undergrowth with the pushchair and hide, crouched down. I try to stay as quiet as possible, hardly breathing, but my heart is pounding as I hear them approach. They're back on the road. 'English? English, where are you?' they're yelling. They can speak English, which amazes me, but with an accent that's not Russian. I fear I've broken some branches and they'll see this and follow me. *But they run past. They keep on going.*

I can't believe I've got away. I've escaped. I keep seeing shadows among the trees, but they don't come back. *Get a grip*, I say to myself. *Eat something, get a rest.* Nothing like this has happened before, or will necessarily happen again. It's fear that is the enemy. I have to deal with incidents like this and put them behind me.

I know I've cared about succeeding on this run more than anything on earth, especially after my visit to Kitezh, and also because not long ago was Clive's birthday, 10 April. It occurs to me that I would never have done anything so dangerous when he was alive. He would have been so worried, yet I still believe he would have been for the run, in light of all that happened.

The most significant thing about leaving Moscow is that I have 7117km to run just to get to the end of Siberia. I have to get through as much as I can before next winter and temperatures of –50°C in that region. So now, while the weather is good, my run becomes a race. Thanks to the new buggy and not having a load on my back I've even sometimes managed up to 40km a day. And I've fallen in love with this part of Russia in the same disarming way that places like Tower Hamlets mean more during the London Marathon. You belong to places where you go as a runner. Perhaps it's effort that makes everything vivid.

On 11 April, Easter Sunday, I run through ancient Vladimir which, around AD 920, was the capital of Russia, and visit the cathedral, eat Easter eggs dyed blue with the juice of berries. I carry on past villages with brightly painted wooden houses, elderly people sitting in the porches with buckets of berries, and eggs and others things put out for sale. About 200km after this, approaching Nizhniy Novgorod, poor Columbine gets a puncture with twenty thorns in one tyre, but that's OK, because though I haven't been able to buy enough patches, a man who owns a local tractor factory fixes Columbine up a treat, to the loud cheering of his staff.

Soon it's May. There are many more people in the forests now, because the weather is good, and also many mosquitoes. Most folk are collecting berries and mushrooms and look like ghouls wrapped in white muslin against the mossies. I can imagine how all the fairy stories, myths and tales of zombies in this part of the world have come about.

Everybody is unbelievably good to me. I meet no more nasty men, though many interesting ones. Close to the Tartarstan border en route to the Ural mountains two delightful old gentleman during a downpour take a lot of trouble teaching me the art of lighting a fire, even in the rain, with bits of bark and so on. Just before I leave them they inform me they're murderers on the run, but it's been a big mistake and a long time ago.

Then on the road I meet a gang of roadworkers on their way east to break stones. They all have metal teeth, which I'm told is quite fashionable in these parts owing to the expense of anything else. They're so nice, insisting I have one of their loaves of bread.

Kazan, the beautiful ancient city of the Tartars standing on seven hills like Rome, has always been proud and independent. Apparently Lenin was here as a student and got temporarily evicted for being troublesome. I stay in a hotel as a treat and while cleaning my stove burn a little hole in the carpet. I'm mortified, but hotel staff are so kind. I ask them up to inspect it and they measure up the little inch of the hole, only charging me 2000 roubles, roughly £20, saying it would be no bother to patch it invisibly.

The only downside is that shoes despatched by Saucony haven't arrived via DHL yet. Back on the road again, thinking my old ones will do for now, I find the heels are suddenly wearing down very fast because of the hard road instead of soft snow, and the extra high mileage. I'm a clumsy runner and tend to run unevenly, and the heels have worn down like ski slopes. But on the road again a car draws up and a gentleman gets out, saying he's a chiropractor and has a solution. I give him 200 roubles and he speeds off, returning with a pair of blue carpet slippers which were all he's been able to get from a village shop. He puts the Saucony insoles into the slippers, saying that like this I'll be flat and balanced evenly. I run like that for many hundreds of kilometres.

The landscape has changed. The nodding donkeys of oilfield areas have become forests again. I'm exceptionally tired one night and, finding a peaceful place in the woods, fall asleep. I wake up to hear running footsteps crunching on the old leaves that still cover the forest floor among the new wild flowers and undergrowth. The scene looks fearful. A man is rushing straight at me in the bright moonlight waving an axe, his white face set and clenched. He seems to be shouting with anger. I'm stuck. My bivvi is up and my kit unpacked, the little buggy folded.

I can't run away fast this time so I stay still and shout, 'Hello, how are you? I love Russia,' or something like that. It makes no difference. He keeps coming. I jump out and find my faithful slippers which are all I still have and I don't fancy doing a sprint in them. Then all at once I realise he's not shouting with fury after all, he's yelling with joy. He grabs me as I stand there stunned and envelops me in a friendly but overwhelming Russian hug. It's a respectful hug, even though his axe almost cuts my ear off by mistake. He says his name is Alexei and that he's a woodsman and explains that he and some of his friends have been having a vodka party a little distance off that began some hours ago. He's never seen a woman sleeping on her own in the forest before and declares I'm definitely the woman for him, but when I say I'm spoken for he's quite gallant. He invites me to the party but I decline, saying I'm tired, it's 1am. Then he just smiles very kindly and says, well, he and his friends will toast me and all my family. He speaks gently and slowly for the sake of my pidgin Russian.

I don't feel afraid of him in any way and the fear in my heart ever since the men chased me is all at once gone. He's given me a sense of peace and actually looked more frightening to start with than he might have been otherwise, as I had seen by the light of my torch that his axe had blood on it. But it was his own blood. The poor man cut his hand in the excitement. He lets me disinfect the cut with some vodka and a little of my iodine, and I bandage it for him. Then he departs with many good wishes. I'm asleep again before I know it.

In the morning, when I wake later than expected, spiders have woven little webs around the guy ropes of my tiny home and the wild flowers grow in a glorious array of purple, lacy white and yellow with tall, spiky purple thistles; the saplings even seem to have grown an inch during the night. Summer doesn't happen in Russia, it explodes.

I think I may have imagined the woodsman Alexei. Then I see the parcel. It contains sausage, bread and a small bottle of vodka. He's written a note in a rough hand in Cyrillic. It says, *'For Rosie!'*

Only in this part of Russia, I think, could you meet a man with an axe in the forest in the middle of the night with it ending up as a positive experience.

CHAPTER 18

Running into Asia

Russia, May–June 2004

'The last freedom,' says Sergey, a man with sunken blue eyes, 'is inner freedom. One does not *ever* have to give it up. I have fought to keep mine. How old do you think I am?'

'Around 65?'

'I'm 30,' he replies, looking at me kindly and self-mockingly. He tells me as we wheel our carts, his ancient one wobbly and full of mushrooms, that he was brought up along the Techa river near Chelyabinsk and suffered radiation sickness. He says the ground is still radioactive there to this day. But he hopes now to get better, go to university and become a doctor.

I listen to him with awe as we walk down the far side of the Ural mountains, towards the next town on my route which is actually Chelyabinsk. The Urals, with their green peaceful forests and scarlet butterflies as large as your hand, make such a contrast to the film I had once seen about the nearby Techa region. The atomic weapons complex called Mayak is situated 80km north of Chelyabinsk on the banks of the Techa River. Allegedly radioactive waste has been systemically dumped into this river, and people who live along the banks, and whose only water supply it is, have received an average of 'four times more radiation than those affected by Chernobyl', it's said, though this was not admitted for years. Many people got sick with cancer and other illnesses and didn't know why.

Sergey says he got off lightly and wants to go back to help. Before he heads back into the woods to continue gathering, he assures me that everything is fine in this part of the Urals, that's why they come here to get berries and mushrooms, and he also gives me a beautiful large log he's carved and painted. 'It's a gift so you'll remember Techa.'

I somehow stick it into my cart and tie it on, promising I'll send it home when I next can and keep for ever, and mean it. Running towards Siberia, I think about all the suffering there and how it's still going on in so many ways. As I continue through the mountains, the people in small dwellings by the roadside never seem to stop working, clearing the patches of land, sowing seeds, fabricating little plastic coverings so they can grow tomatoes, and always making jokes as they smile and call out to me.

When the fiercest, biggest mosquitoes in the world descend, they say things like, 'You don't need the KGB to have more bugs than you can handle around here.' It's so unexpected the way people talk so much to me, perhaps to practise their English. Or because I don't speak Russian at all well, though learning some each day, they feel they can talk to me more freely. Or maybe the feeling I have of belonging to them is in the way of travelling: I'm alone, I'm not a threat, as if the way of travelling is a pathway in itself. Or maybe I just fit in along with the mushroom gatherers.

At length a smart BMW draws up and the driver, who says he's from Moscow, actually asks me for directions. I have my head in a scarf and am wearing long trousers as I've run out of mosquito repellent. He's taken me for a local person.

'You are from England?' he says, astounded. 'Well, you should be told that the Russian people after Communism have become lazy. They won't help themselves.'

Before I can retort he zooms off again.

I'm running through the land, on the periphery of the life here, but he's made me very angry. Especially because the next 'vehicle' I see is a wheelchair. Hailing me with shouts, coming the other way towards me, a pretty girl with dark hair and elfin features pushes the wheelchair, with a young man sitting in it.

'I'm Lara,' she says. 'We're heading north, to find help, and find work.'

She leaves her friend with me while she darts off into the woods. He can speak no English, talks no Russian to me at all, but grins and suddenly takes hold of the bars on the outside of the chair's wheels and spins his wheelchair round and round like a top, as if he wants to make me laugh, and he does. I'll never forget him or his example – if you've nothing else to give, you give yourself instead and make a smile happen.

Lara emerges with mosquitoes clinging to her face, clutching brushwood. 'We're going to make a little fire,' she declares gaily in English, inviting me to have tea with them. 'Everything is going to be fine for us.' She explains that her boyfriend has cancer. They lost their house, because although the hospital visits and doctors' diagnoses were free of charge, they'd had to pay for medicines by taking out a loan on the little house they bought at the beginning of capitalism. Now they have no money at all, not even for the medicine, but her brother lives in Moscow and can get the treatment for him. They are walking there or hitching if they can.

One of the lorries carrying cars to Kazakhstan stops and presses a wad of money into the man's hands and is gone, before any of us can say anything to him. It just breaks me up how people here, just like at home, help one another, and here it's all much harder. It reminds me how hard Clive's fight was with so much more help than this. I give my money too, which isn't much. Then I run for Chelyabinsk.

As I finally reach Asia, it's a huge moment; I descend from the Urals, leaving European Russia behind for ever. Same country, different continent.

After all I've heard about Chelyabinsk, to arrive in this city, completely closed to all foreigners, and to most Russians from other parts until 1992, spooks me. It's like other cities I've passed through that sit like islands amidst Russia's wilderness, quite a pleasant place nowadays. With banks, shops, offices, even a DHL office from which I collect my shoes, saying goodbye to the carpet slippers and the ill-fitting volleyball shoes a kind man gave me en route. One other bright spot is a bike shop where I get Columbine repaired. The best moment of all is meeting up with Linda Cross, the British Consul from Yekaterinburg quite a distance away, who's driven many kilometres just to take coffee with me, in an Irish pub of all things called the Fox and Goose. She makes me chuckle, sticking her head around the door, and singing, 'Rosie, I presume!'

She makes my day when, among much else, she takes into her safekeeping Sergey's painted log which, though beautiful, is heavy. She vows to send it safely to my home in Wales even by diplomatic bag if no other secure way can be found.

Alone again, Chelyabinsk is depressing. Not many children around and I'm told that people have until recently been afraid to have children, as so many are born with health problems, probably due to the radiation to the north. The population is plummeting: the average life expectancy in Chelyabinsk is 58 and falling. There are all the goodies in the world in the shops but because of inflation pensioners receive just enough to buy a week's worth of food. Although the gangsters (called 'New Russians') are doing OK, I'm told, teachers and doctors still earn only US$40 a month. People grow all they can in every spot of wasteland around the city that becomes converted into vegetable or market gardens of some kind. They survive as cheerfully as they can, but in every sense life here is unspeakably hard.

I think about the apparent normality of life here: the shiny shops and parks are perhaps a kindlier, but just as effective, way of hiding the reality of Chelyabinsk as the guns, guards and barbed wire across the river banks once had been.

I don't seek to find the worst, or abuse the fact that I'm running across Russia because the authorities have granted permission, but I'm determined to tell the truth about how wonderful Russian people seem to be, despite everything. I've found that I care as deeply about this as I do about succeeding, and I don't care about anything else that might happen to me.

As I set off across the western Siberian plains, I sometimes think, I shall never get out of Russia. I'll be in Siberia for the rest of my life.

But how lucky I am to be here and to be free. I *will* make it.

CHAPTER 19

Omsk: The First Race

Siberia, June–September 2004

I'm running in a fury. I get bolder at sleeping beside the road instead of going into the forest. This way, I can run about 15km, rest in the bivvi, then be on my way again quickly, hoping my legs have forgotten all about the distance. Last year I flew 6000 miles to run the Siberian Marathon in Omsk for the Railway Hospital. I'm determined to be on the start-line on 7 August, this time after having run there.

I've been trying out new techniques with food. The staple is *grescu* which is cheap and three handfuls make a meal. I can cook it by boiling for ten minutes, eat it with a little sugar for breakfast and flavouring cube in it for lunch or dinner. I also buy local produce like a cabbage if I can get it. I drink water from streams because I have a filter bottle. I'm healthy and strong. I've learnt that you don't have to have everything you like all the time. I remember that Somerset Maugham said that writing is achieved by what you don't put in and I'm feeling more and more that running long distance is all about what you don't carry.

It's only 770km from Chelyabinsk to Omsk, There should be plenty of time, but I have to run through 150km north of Kazakhstan en route to get the exit and entry stamps in my passport that are the requirements of my multi-entry Russian visa; and it's possible there'll be delays at the borders.

I run mostly through the wilderness, crossing into Kazakhstan without hitches on 25 June. I do a sprint finish to the border post, and the officials just clap and wave me through.

Fields with swaying tall grass, silvery in the sunshine, and summer green forests stretch away as far as the eye can see. It's very remote. Along the road that gleams with lakes that are mirages in the heat, there are beautiful wild roses and purple flowers like Welsh campion, and iridescent dragonflies whirring like miniature helicopters, and black clouds and swarms of mosquitoes. In contrast to the beauty, each time I awake after a rest to continue my run, there's a scene straight out of a sci-fi horror movie. The bugs whirr and hover viciously over a large, wriggling cocoon, which is the bivvi; with me inside it struggling to get insect repellent on all parts of my body before going out to be amongst them. It's sweltering hot and sticky. I run in shorts as I can't bear not to. As advised by locals, I pour half a bottle of vodka over my legs, which eases the bites and prevents infection, but it doesn't put off the mosquitoes. They are definitely not teetotallers.

On 2 July I'm back in Russia again with a bang! The officials almost kiss me. I think they're sorry for me, so sweaty and covered in bites and bumps. On 1 July I'm only 137km from Omsk. It's tough-going with a headwind, and I have little to eat. I've run out of buckwheat. I keep in mind that I'm not far from my friends in Omsk now and know they're looking to see me.

There's 'mossiemania' now – worse than the Kazakstani ones. And they *love* the repellent with their dinners; they can't get enough of it. The only relief is when the lorries roar past on this busier part of the road and spray me with grit and dust which is quite a relief as the mossies get swept away in the slipstream … but they catch up. It's all worth it, though, and so exciting reaching Omsk on 6 July. I run across the big bridge of the Irtysh River into town.

'I've got back, I've got back.' I hear it in my footsteps and am almost shouting it aloud. None of my plans could have matched the way it's turned out. I'm thrilled beyond expression, that after everything I've made it nearly a month to the day before the marathon. In spite of my efforts I haven't gone very fast, and had two slow days because of a twisted ankle, but I guess as Steven Seaton has always said, 'You only have to think of the next step. Big distances are just many little steps all joined up.'

Elena, my friend, marathon organiser, teacher, tour guide, among other jobs, is the same as ever. Her hair short, tufted like a fair-haired Judy Garland. She's wearing a bright pink T-shirt, a gift I later learn from her best friend in England. On it is written, 'I'm the girl your parents warned you about!' She's rushed to meet me and scolds me for not getting there even sooner, as I managed to call her on the rickety mobile a few days ago. She'd made special home-made soup and chocolate pudding that's been waiting for me since then. She drags me off to stay with her. It's the only place I've not just run towards but back to. It's my Siberian home.

The crumbling building stands like a bleak block of concrete. The tiny, neat, well-organised flat Elena shares with her daughter Laura, the bright carpets, pictures, comfy sofa, old computer are all the same as last time. Their long-haired, green-eyed marmalade cat Ryzha recognises me, jumping on my knees and purring. Between them, they spoil and fuss over me.

I email family and friends on Elena's computer. They can also phone me halfway around the world. Eve often says, 'Mum, there's a circle of hands all around the world bringing you home to us.'

It's agreed that as the summer is so short and I'm lucky to have got to Omsk early, I can continue my run eastwards for a few weeks and then make a mark on the map to return to, before getting a lift back to Omsk for the race.

I set off at 5am on 10 July. It's an easy run for the next 575km to Novorsibersk. I see hay-making in fields between forests; rose hips by the side of the road so I can make tea with them; two bears shuffling thoughtfully across the road but taking no notice of me; black ears sticking up above bushes for a while and then disappearing. The next time I stop, there's scuffling around the bivvi. I peep out and spot them, but they are still not bothering about me: they're busily grazing the blueberries around my camping spot. They aren't large – maybe the size of six-month-old calves, but powerful in frame, with big claws and thick dark fur, and little eyes and sloping shoulders that don't quite seem real, though they are very much so. I hold my breath then relax: nothing happens.

I'm delayed this morning because it doesn't seem wise to disturb them as it may anger them. So I wait until they eventually move away. I decide it's better in future not to camp on their blueberry 'dining tables' in the forest. Pretty inconsiderate of me and I didn't mean it. I know I have to get used to not being unnerved by bears and to 'acclimatise' to them, or I might as well give up my run right now.

I make it to Novorsibirsk ('New Siberia'), happy to have 575km more of my world course under my belt before the marathon. Some of Elena's friends drive me back to Omsk with Columbine. It's the buggy's finest hour. The Race Director says he'll only allow me to enter the race if I push it all the way around the course as it's now famous in Russia. I stand there on the start-line on 7 August, clutching the pushchair handles. It's got the backpack on it and also a teddy bear and charity banners.

The gun fires, a band plays, the crowds shout out loud cheers, and I'm off among 7500 other runners. There are 1000 in the marathon, the others being in a 5km and relay marathon all starting at the same time.

A child rushes out from the crowd, jumping onto the pushchair. The mother follows to collect him, but then smiling and shrugging, decides to join him and runs the race with me instead. The onlookers throw flowers at all the runners, and are roaring and waving us along. The whole of Omsk is standing there in the sunshine.

Steven Seaton, editor of *Runner's World*, has flown over from Britain to run the race and support me, as has Geoff, whose first overseas marathon Omsk was when he and I were the only British runners last year. So there are three British runners this year among a host of competitors from every former Soviet republic and others far and wide. It brings all kinds of emotions and lumps to my throat. I haven't seen anyone from home for so long. They've come to run with me but I've urged them ahead. I'm definitely in the 'just getting around' class.

It's a pleasant two-loop marathon course through the city and along the river, and there's the most extraordinary atmosphere. Many onlookers have stood all day in the scorching Siberian sun, and most have brought water for the runners. It's great of them to make sure the runners are OK between the official watering stations, I keep thinking how Elena and other people here still have to filter their water for three days before it's safe to drink because of the toxins in the otherwise clean river from old ex-Soviet factories upstream. Some people are holding out beakers of tea and small cakes. I can't get over how generous Omsk citizens are in the midst of their difficulties.

I'm discovering the slower the runner in the race the greater the fuss you get. There's more time for people to grab you aside for a moment, shake your hand, shove bunches of flowers in your arms. I'm given a bunch of orange blooms I had on the pushchair for several miles before giving them away to an old lady who looked as though she'd like them. I'd also collected several more children who jump on and off the buggy, alternating between riding and running with me. I'm the Pied Piper! I realise about 10km from the end that I'll *never* make it. I'm running out of time after all this, as the marathon limit is five hours.

I bolt for the finish line with a group of children racing in with me, one still perched precariously on top of the rucksack in the buggy. We make it in 5 hours, 7 minutes, 30 seconds. But the Race Director decides that, calculating the way you do with a horse that's had to race taking extra weight along, I've made it OK. I give my medal to the children.

We've made it after all and it's the end of an era – Columbine's last run. I'll never forget the great help I've had from the UK, and always when I needed it the most.

Steven, some time ago when he learned that Columbine was getting frail, had commissioned a new cart/sled for the Siberian winter for me from Steve Holland and Giles Dyson, who make equipment for Sir Ranulph Fiennes to use on his polar expeditions. Thanks to Geoff arranging its transport with DHL, the new cart is already here in Omsk, waiting to be collected and unwrapped.

I soon understand why, when Geoff mentioned coming out, he talked about 'the three of us', meaning the cart as well. It's a character, big, tough and strong, with shafts, so I can pull it as if I were the pony, and Sir Ranulph himself has kindly donated the grand red harness I'll wear. Hercules, as I call my cart, has been built of iron and fibreglass, because he can be welded and mended if he gets broken or into trouble, in a way that would be difficult in Siberia with an aluminium buggy. 'The trolley', as his designers simply call him, is basically a cart with two wheels that can be taken off in deep snow to become a sled.

My buggy Columbine will always be loved and cherished. I send her home via DHL to Tenby and will keep her for ever. She'll probably be writing a book of her own about her adventures, but she'd never be able to hold all the equipment for the winter. I'm so grateful to have the new cart and to have been reunited at Omsk with the satphone and solar panel, as there's plenty of room in Hercules.

Along with Hercules I take transport back to my mark on the map at Novorsibersk, and on 11 August set off boldly to run eastwards.

There's a big psychological boost in having run the extra miles before the marathon, and be ahead of myself, but 4800km of Siberia still have to be covered. No use at all just taking small steps now. I have to think of it as giant steps, as '1000km footsteps'.

Winter is coming. I have to live through it and keep going. With Hercules I hope I can. He's heavy to pull but sturdy and I just have to go for it.

Everything goes well through September as it gradually gets colder. In mountainous, spectacular Krasnoyarsk I have a delightful couple of days when my friend and marathon coach Mike Rowland comes all the way from Newport, laden with the new down clothes generously sponsored by PHD, as I still have such a fear of the cold ahead. In the town's main square we ride horses for hire with fringes on their forelocks.

The weather is worsening and with October comes the first snow. Hercules is doing well: it's much easier to pull than push. I'm running through the wilderness, and gradually making progress.

The satphone is a treasured link to the world, mostly used for sending and receiving short emails. I eke out the batteries because of the cost to my sponsors who've been generous enough. I don't often get it out along the roadside, but today's my birthday and I'm sitting beside Hercules on a deserted road, reading emails from home with tears of joy and sorrow. The lonely feeling of missing home – I mean the people I love more than a physical place – never leaves me. I still don't know how long I'll be running.

A man appears in view, riding a bicycle laden with baskets. He slows down and stops. I'm pleased to see him as he's selling small sweet Siberian apples, recently on the trees and a big treat. Next day he comes back and gets off the bike, standing beside me.

'I have to have your phone,' he says quietly, almost in a hiss.

I look down at his right hand. He's holding a stiletto knife, and it's pointed right at my heart.

CHAPTER 20

Bandit on a Bicycle

Siberia, October 2004

His hand is shaking violently; the blade of the knife rips my jacket. He starts screaming and shouting and I have to escape. I *have* to escape. I can't run. He can get me before I run.

I'm not collapsing in a blur. My mind is trying to save me. Easy ... easy. You can't let it get to you until you've got away. Instinct says that, amidst everything in the turmoil of my head, to move suddenly would be the most dangerous thing to do. Then in an instant I see the man shuddering, not because he's crazy but because he himself is terrified. Maybe he's desperate, maybe he's as unused to holding people up as I am to having it done to me, but I can feel the point of the knife on my skin. I think, *Talk to him. I know I have to talk to him. That's the way.*

I say something in Russian like, 'Don't do this. Don't be stupid ... I'm a *babouska* ... I have a grandson!'

Suddenly, by instinct or impulse, certainly not because I'm brave, I push his knife away. He stares at me in horror as if I have some secret weapon and begins to cry as well as shout. I'm shocked. He leaps on his bicycle, spilling all the little red apples, and pedals furiously away. At last I sink to my knees in fear. He hasn't got the phone.

Yet for all that, I think: he isn't evil, just poor, wretched and tempted. He's not like the men in the red and yellow shirts. I'm unscathed. It's just as good now as if it hadn't happened at all.

If I stay positive, with a clear brain, adopt caution and action instead of worry and fear, that's the way through moments like this. How lucky I am to breathe, to be able to see and run and live. It really would be unreasonable if, alone in wild parts of the world, I were never attacked. It's only happened once before, and ended up fine. I've met 10,000 kindly people in between. I must keep them in mind. Negative thoughts and fears that cloud the mind are the real danger. Being positive isn't being unrealistic, it's the way to look plainly at what's happening and deal with the dangers. I decide to call him my 'Bandit on a Bicycle'.

I'm proceeding eastwards parallel to the Trans-Siberian Railway but it's not often in sight as the snowy undergrowth near the track is impenetrable. The trains, if I glimpse them, are like long grey snowy monsters roaring by in clouds of snow spray that beat up from the tracks. Any dreams I've had of passengers waving, or even throwing food to me, are soon dismissed as fantasy. What does happen, which I never expected, is that the starlings, who back home in Tenby can imitate the blackbird's beautiful song in a way that's uncanny, in this part of Siberia actually imitate the sound of trains, going *'Chuff, chuff, chuff'* or something similar. It's part of forest life and at first quite startling.

On hilltops all I see is forest, stretching into infinity. Siberia is a place of darkness and light. The half moon and stars shine through the forest trees as if the clear night will never end, but by daylight when it's snowing you can see little further than the snowflakes on the end of your nose. Other times it goes back to rain, a solid torrent as if all 336 rivers flowing into Lake Baikal, still several hundred kilometres to the east, had ended up in the heavens here and burst their banks.

The wolves aren't around yet. All the bears seem to have gone to sleep; but there's a different type of wildlife about. When I crawl in and out of the bivvi, ticks get in somehow and bite me as enthusiastically as the mosquitoes had. If I dab Vaseline on the ticks, they're smothered well enough to drop out of my skin, but they're nasty little fellows with bloated bodies and horrible, wriggling little black legs and hard to reach on the back of my neck.

Other creatures making the most of getting as much to eat as possible are the cheeky forest mice with golden fur and bright eyes. They're everywhere right now, dashing up and down the trees and over the forest floor, collecting nuts or seeds. They're quite unafraid, and often just sit outside in the snow, looking for scraps and even trying to get in with me. I think they've not seen a human before, and don't know what I am. They have a taste for my buckwheat and I learn to leave a bit of grain outside the flap as 'rent' since I'm using *their* forest – and because otherwise they might chew their way in to get it. They're like my little cabaret artists and always make me laugh.

*   *   *

Geoff emails on the satphone. He and Inna are flying to Irkutsk and will drive out and find me. Even if I had a shiny back-up jeep, huge budget and big team always on the road, I couldn't have better support. He also makes mysterious comments about belatedly celebrating my birthday.

11 October: a red letter day. Rain pelts down, treetops are bent by the wind and branches moan. It's a lonely part of the road, but suddenly the rain eases and into view, amidst endless forest, a petrol station and 'Kafe' appear as if especially for me. It's the first cafe or sign of a shop I've seen for many days. I don't want to miss Geoff and Inna, but I *have* to go into this place – it's an unwritten law in Siberia, never pass up a chance to buy something to eat. So I put Hercules beside the road in a prominent spot, with the big Welsh flag draped over him, just as Geoff and Inna draw up in their four-wheel hire car from Irkutsk.

The cafe has customers coming in and out; a lady conscientiously washes the floor, even though every footstep makes a new puddle. The little place serves neither tea nor coffee, just cold drinks and some food, but it's warm and friendly and so great to see Geoff and Inna. They've brought a birthday cake from Ann in Tenby; presents from my family and friends; drawings by my two-year-old grandson Michael better than anything by Michelangelo; a photo of Catherine and Nedd. I'm in tears. Also, friends who wish to remain anonymous have sent money to my bank account at home to help my journey expenses, though I never asked for or expected this. Terra Nova has sent a Quasar extreme weather tent; Saucony provides tough trail shoes; and Geoff and Inna have personally bought a replacement for my worn-out stove

During the party, after being alone on the road for so long, I've lost my voice and can hardly speak, which nobody will ever believe. I can only croak my thanks but manage to tell them I feel fine.

'You only look 40 but you sound 86,' remarks Geoff gallantly.

'You look as fresh as if you've only run around the block,' Inna adds.

We have just a few hours together. We cling to each other, then they're gone, back to Irkutsk, 300km away, to catch their flight home.

My voice stays lost: I have a sore throat and fever over the next week. It hurts to breathe and my legs, even after just a few kilometres, become like jelly. I put it down to tick bites and start taking the soggy year-old antibiotics the SOS Clinic in Moscow gave me in case this happened. The clinic inoculated me against the fatal disease that ticks apparently carry, but provided the medicine as they said you can still catch a fever from the ticks.

I must have more of the fever than I realised. I put the wrong PIN in the satphone three times and the word BLOCKED flashes up. I'm isolated, out of touch. I decide to keep going on slowly until I find a person or place with a phone. Vehicles occasionally pass by as if in a different world, probably assuming I'm OK. I don't want to flag down a motorist or get a lift into town or leave Hercules, because I don't know what will happen then or if I can ever get back to continue. Anyway I might as well feel ill and be going somewhere than be ill and not go anywhere at all.

My logbook entries are bleak: *'Go easy. Just get your breath back! Every kilometre is worth it ... A whole kilometre without stopping!'* Next day it's 2km, then 8km. *'Bitter wind ... half-buried in snow.'*

Gradually I get stronger and at last on 23 October reach Irkutsk. When I call home, I find that the message I gave to a man who stopped his car has been emailed to my family. Everyone has my news and is concerned. The unblocking of the satphone is being sorted.

The old houses have eaves carved like wooden lace. Some of the clothes here are very individual too. Men wear flat caps, rather like those worn in Ireland, though with thick scarves around their necks as it's getting snowy and cold. It seems different from any other Russian city; both the older and the new bustling town have a cosmopolitan almost independent spirit. You can understand why Irkutsk held out for three years against the Russian Revolution before being captured. I have a good rest for a few days in a cheap hotel, with Hercules parked in the foyer.

I feel great affection for Hercules: we've made it through our first difficult time together. I still don't feel 100%, but I'm not sick enough to visit a doctor. I think I'm on the mend from the ticks. Keeping going has always been the best medicine ...

On 29 October I set off again led on by the knowledge that Lake Baikal, 'Gem of Siberia' and deepest lake in the world, is only 40km away, though it won't be in sight for a long time yet. My route leads to the southern part of the lake by way of Shelekhov, the next town I reach. Snow is falling thickly. The temperature is –20 but I feel fine, as I'm wearing my down jacket with hood tightly drawn. I'm plodding along happily, pulling Hercules through deep unploughed snow by the side of the road, when suddenly I begin feeling very dizzy.

I open my eyes to see I'm lying on the ground and there's blood on the snow. Then I fall unconscious again.

CHAPTER 21

In a Siberian Hospital

Siberia, November 2004

'You're a very fortunate young lady to have been knocked down by the bus,' the doctor kindly says, 'otherwise you would not have been brought here so we could treat your double pneumonia.'

My head is spinning and I'm trying to focus. All I can think is, *How nice to be called a young lady when you're 86*, because I definitely feel 86 now. I regain consciousness in a crowded hospital corridor. To my surprise Hercules is there too. The pain in my head is terrible. I try to explain that I haven't been feeling very well for a while. The doctor says the antibiotics I took for the tick bite have masked the pneumonia, but X-rays have shown both lungs half-filled with fluid, triggered by the cold. He thinks I've managed to go as far as I have during the past weeks due to my extra lung capacity because I'm so fit. He remarks cheerily that pneumonia isn't always serious but mine is because in a week or two it will be −50°C.

'If you're not cured before then you'll soon be dead,' he adds.

The cuts to my head need five stitches, but they're superficial. I thank the thick hood of my PHD jacket for saving me from worse.

If I'd chosen which bus driver should be the one to run me over I couldn't have picked a lovelier man than Genia. He's here, almost in tears. It wasn't his fault. I'd been weaving all over the road before getting hit, as my temperature was 102°. It was he who'd brought Hercules to the hospital and also had my kit packed into black plastic bags; The passengers had carefully searched for it in the snow. I later discover that not a single item has been lost. There can't be greater testimony to the total honesty and good nature of people around here. I'm very pleased that a lady teacher who speaks perfect English arrives with a policeman to whom I'm able to give a clear statement that no blame is involved, because otherwise Genia might have lost his job.

I'm sent by ambulance from the local hospital to the Pulmonary Department of Irkutsk Regional Hospital and Hercules is taken away by Genia to have his bent shafts straightened. Hercules is a hero: he's protected my equipment by capsizing over it during the crash. Genia says he's going to make him good as new.

My treatment is two big injections in my bottom twice a day. I share a ward with five other women with similar problems. Ward 704, with its greyish walls and wooden bedsteads, seems dark and gloomy, but it's spotlessly clean, and the doctors and nurses show such love and care. The treatment for me, as for Russian patients, is fabulous. The nurses, in smart blue uniforms with watches at their waists and thermometers and pens in their starched top pockets, are as ruthless with the jabs as they are kind in other ways. I have half an hour a day in a grey sack tent on the hospital's top floor that turns out to be an oxygen tent. They put poultices on my legs that have also taken a knock and got bruised. In addition, when I look in the small washroom adjoining the ward, I discover I have a brand new green hairdo, to complement my black eye.

This is because they've treated my stitches with the economical universally acclaimed *espiritu*, emerald-green disinfectant, often used in Russia for the treatment of chickenpox, giving children green spots, and it's spread through my hair.

I start getting better. Natasha, in the next bed, begins to revive at the same time and gives me intensive Russian lessons. I can soon count to nearly 1000 and she insists on telling me an English poem she's learnt: *'Mother, father, sister, brother, hand in hand with one another ...'* which soon drives everyone crazy.

Not only do I have my friends in the ward, but the policeman who took my statement, his two little daughters, the English teacher Arina, Genia, his wife and brothers, all come to visit me every day.

The chief doctor, Tatyana Rastompakhova, has decided I caught the pneumonia virus maybe as far back as Omsk as I had done the marathon and run hard without a long rest since then, and not eaten enough in her view. She puts me on a diet of lumps of fat with my semolina for breakfast each day, and soon I'm as strong as a pony.

There is a canteen with bread, tea, soup, semolina and a special type of thick porridge and the *sala* fat among other items on the menu. I have an abiding memory of what a progressive, benevolent place Irkutsk Hospital truly is. The doctors explain that this hospital uses generic antibiotics and other fairly inexpensive treatments. Therefore unlike in many Russian hospitals, both treatment and food are free to Russian and Siberian patients, though foreigners have to pay.

I'm happy to pay after all they've done for me, but am a little anxious about the cost as they seem to have done every possible health check, thoroughly testing my heart, liver and every single part of my body. I made the big mistake of thinking my insurance was valid for two years, but it's recently run out, only covering me for one year. But the whole bill is roughly £100. I double-check in case they've been lenient with me, but it's the full cost, and thanks to Ann who's got a new bank card to me in Irkutsk via DHL, I can use an ATM that I found along a corridor and pay the hospital direct. Though the signal is poor, I have been able to call her and my family on the satphone.

After eight days in hospital, Genia comes to collect me, smiling from ear to ear, and takes me to stay with his mother-in-law to prepare for the road. The first thing I notice when we arrive at her little red and green painted dacha is Hercules sitting in the snowy courtyard, all mended and raring to go. It's suddenly much colder. Icicles hang from the cabin's roof and the snow is deep except where a path has been shovelled to the entrance.

Inside everything is warm and cosy. There is a smell of baking, children's drawings bedeck the walls and a little wooden clock chimes the hour as I walk inside. Galina, a lively elderly lady with bright blue eyes in a strong, sculpted face, is waiting for me with many grandchildren and other members of the family. On the lacy cloth spread out on the table is a delightful feast of cakes, fish, pickled berries, jams and other things. I stay here for two days and I'll never be able to think of Galina without picturing all her grandchildren crowding into her small dwelling. She is much loved. I tell Galina – as I do everyone – the reasons for my journey.

Everybody puts concerted efforts into helping me prepare for my run in the cold. Genia says I'm right to keep going, as many of the swamps and bridgeless rivers further east might only be negotiable while they remained frozen hard. Genia, his wife Natasha and Galina and the others air my warm sleeping-bags and clothes, and everything is carefully packed so it fits neatly into my cart. The battle against winter will be won with a mixture of high-tech PHD down clothing and equipment and local lore and advice. The big boots I bought some time ago are rejected: I always find them cold as the sweat from running freezes in them. And I'm not often going to be under the roof of a house to dry them beside a fire. Instead, Genia lines my trail shoes with fur, weatherproofing them with varnish and making little gaiters for them, thus creating footwear that's brilliantly warm yet light, like the moccasins that the Yakutian people wear year round further east. Also, on friends' recommendation, in the town's market I buy *velinkis* – felt Wellingtons – that all villagers wear in winter, I'm told, and which would be good for early morning or evening, or just for plodding about in the snow.

Best of all, Galina advises me to eat a lot of garlic to strengthen my lungs. I try it right away and it seems to help when I go for a practice run. She also says I need to keep a clove of garlic in my pocket and hold it to my face in a hand-kerchief from time to time, breathing in the aroma. That will keep the lungs healthier and keep infections at bay, as well as frightening off the Siberian vampires.

Arina takes me back to the local hospital to have the last of my stitches removed and to thank the doctors who first looked after me. I'm also invited to give a talk at the Lyceum where Arina teaches. I'm not allowed to talk Russian. She wants her students to practise their English.

'Bread in your pocket is one kind of survival in Russia, education is another. Whatever happens in tomorrow's Russia, an educated person will be able to cope better,' she says. 'We've had a hard history, but there's always hope beyond the horizons of despair.'

The students share cake and tea with me and write touch-ing remarks in my book. Iluna, 15, writes, *It's the first time in my life I meet an English woman. I'm glad you love our country Siberia.* Petrova writes, *I am very glad to meet you. I am fond of studying English, French and Latin. I would like to be a translator.*

Next day everybody comes to see me off including Genia, Natasha his wife, and Galina and her grandchildren, bundled up like little bears. It's an emotional moment. I wonder if I'll ever see these people again to whom I owe so much.

It's snowing hard and they're gathered in the snow, smil-ing and waving, I look back again a few minutes later and can hardly see them. They're disappearing in the blizzard yet still standing there, as if it wasn't the snow but a camera that's fading them out – like THE END in a film.

The third time I look, they're gone. I'm alone in a world of white.

Over the next two months temperatures descend to –40 and –50. Nothing matters now except to spend every single moment struggling forwards, and fighting the cold.

CHAPTER 22

Winter in Siberia

Siberia, December 2004–February 2005

Worse than the cold or dangers or anything else, what drives me forward when it's −50 is the fear of the distances still ahead of me. What also drives me forward is that there's no way back. I could go home physically if I put out a call on the satphone, but I can't go back mentally because if I don't finish my run the journey really would never end, and there's so far to go. I've run for over a year and for thousands of miles, yet I feel like someone still on the first mile of the London Marathon. All the biggest battles are in the mind so I bow into the blizzard and keep going.

One of the worst moments is when I receive a message on the satphone to call Eve who tells me that my brother Ronnie has unexpectedly died. I'm extremely sad about it. He was a poet and so I take the opportunity while running past Baikal to pick a white stone from the shore and fling it into the deep waters of the lake. As the stone sinks, I think about him and believe he would have liked this. I pray for Marianne. I get through to her on the phone for a few moments. It's hard to go back for the funeral. Because of the cost, there's a good chance I can't get back on the run, but I cannot put the run ahead of her. I shall never get over that in this time of greatest sorrow for Marianne, it is she who gives me courage.

'Go *on*,' she says. 'Go on for all of us ... You are blessed. Don't forget, I shall be waiting for you at the *finish!*'

By the end of November, Baikal is a long way behind me. I'm running along a lonely icy road and the sheets of snow have kept flattening me. The road seems more like a cold desert than the wilderness either side. Every moment is spent thinking about the cold and how to cope. The biggest weapon is to stop before dark because after darkness it gets much worse. The frightening thing is there's nowhere to go. The slopes down to the woods look steep and dangerous. I carry on, it's getting darker and soon I won't be able to see what lies around me beyond the beam of the torch anyway. Then at last I spy a little hollow. That will have to do. I pitch the tent as quickly as I can. The trickiest time is between when you stop running and when you're safely tucked into the sleeping bags. After that life is just 'household routine'.

People later ask, 'How do you manage to eat? To sleep out in the woods for so long?' And 'How do you wash and go to the toilet?' Women's plumbing is definitely a disadvantage. My adventures with the 'chamber-pot' in the tent would amaze even Houdini but I manage OK, even though I have to wriggle out of seven pairs of thermal bottoms, big down trousers and *four* sleeping bags. Ice covers my possessions, frozen breath hangs in tattered curtains in the air and all the ice crystals shower down on top of me when I move.

There's no bubble bath, but the ziplock bag of snow-water has melted next to me in the night and I can wash my face, hands and other bits in the body-warm water that is the Siberian 'on the road luxury bathroom'. You can do almost anything but have to do it differently here.

Food? I'm eking out a loaf of bread that's frozen solid. I put the bread in the sleeping bags (my Siberian microwave) so that it can thaw enough to eat. If I can get the tiny stove to light, hot food is boiled buckwheat and *sala* fat, as it's possible to carry a month's supply, plus garlic and vitamins. (A friend later says, 'Rosie! please don't write a cookbook! Leave that to Martha or Delia!')

Siberia is the emptiest place on earth. The United States would fit into Siberia without touching any of its boundaries, with 100,000km left over. The loneliness and darkness in a Siberian forest at −50 is beyond words. There are very few hours of daylight. When dawn finally comes, I can see firs, crystal white and deadly cold, in a world that's more exquisite and frightening than anything I've ever known At other times, trees are like phantoms, scarcely visible in the thick snow. At night owls hoot, foxes call, wolves howl eerily, heartstoppingly, in the distance. Nothing matters except the cold. I keep the mitts on one hand and work with the other, swapping round. Without good equipment, the line between somehow managing and losing it, between life and death, is very narrow. My most vivid image is of the people who live in the forest with almost nothing.

I've been told there are homeless men in these mountains who are dangerous and might rob or even murder me, but I haven't seen any and have to go this way anyhow. There's only the wild mountainous road through the forests. One night the snow's so deep I can't pull Hercules far off the verge. I'm putting the tent up when I notice fresh footprints in the snow. A very thin man like a wraith appears, in hardly any clothes for the cold and wearing a hessian sack with ropes as straps forming a backpack. I can now see he's a pleasant old man with deep-etched lines on his face. He says that he and other friends have a camp at the top of the mountain, and I should come. But the path is too steep for Hercules. I give him a little buckwheat and he goes on his way.

I wake to hear a loud slurred voice shouting, *'Come outside, come out ... I want you! I always get obeyed, I am Genghis Khan.'* There's a big rumpus outside and raised voices. As I struggle to put my boots on, I realise what's happened. The homeless men up the mountain have come down – to defend me. They're fighting off the drunken man. I come out, but the drunk has gone by now and the old men of the mountains are smiling. I shall always think of these men. I just can't understand how they have so little and yet survive here and can still help me. What I never expected in Siberia is how the deepest solitude, which you'd think could go on for ever, alternates with vivid images of Siberian people I meet who are so few against the vast landscape, but who will always be so special to me.

The temperature drops to –55°C. On 23 December I write in my log:

I fight to survive or I'll literally be frozen solid. Everything is in the sleeping bag with me. Everything is frozen inside and out. You can forget toothpaste, it's frozen more solid than solid. Best friend is the small knife with which, with effort, I can still hack a few crumbs of bread. Don't give up or you'll be a frozen body. My admiration for Ran Fiennes is unbounded. In Siberia in deep winter today I'm aware that somewhere inside all the layers is me. I can't see my body, haven't seen it for weeks. Just try to look after it. But I WILL win. I AM managing. The shortest day is gone. I've conquered it. Now the days will get longer. However painful and cold – one promise will be kept: the days will get longer!

One of the problems in this cold is that when the soot flies up from the stove it's impossible to keep my down clothes and jacket clean. I worry if I do meet anyone that I might seem disgusting to them or, even worse, frightening. People can naturally be suspicious and the police might even think I'm a criminal.

When things are difficult, something great always happens. When my sorrow about hearing about the death of my brother Ronnie had been at its most raw some weeks ago, Giles Smith of ITV Wales, who lives in Tenby, flew all the way out to find me. Ann Rowell persuaded ITV to come purely, it seemed, so I could be brought letters of support and early Christmas presents. That's the 'Ann Rowell way'. Now, in the middle of the wilds in a village, when I've been so very lucky to find a cafe in which to warm up on Christmas Eve, I hear a voice I know. It turns out to be Natasha.

I met Natasha and Fedor way back near Irkutsk. Natasha, who jumps with both feet in the air with happiness or excitement when she's talking, and serious Fedor, an inventor, have driven 600km so I won't be alone at Christmas. They've saved up the money for the petrol and represent my family. As Eve says in a loving Christmas message on the satphone, 'Don't forget we're here with you – and Natasha and Fedor came for us all.'

The weather is kind: it's only –25°C in a little clearing in the forest. They park their elderly van, decorated with tinsel and silvery bells, and bring delicious food and gifts and some of Fedor's home-made vodka to celebrate. It's in a small bottle but even diluted six times it's the strongest vodka I've ever tasted. We sleep very well tonight. During the whole year-and-a-half-run so far, nobody has stayed out in the forest through the night with me before. It means so much.

So many nights under the stars in forest clearings and on mountain-sides in the next few months. The loneliness, this immensity somehow contrast with the people who always support me. On New Year's Eve I see figures standing by the roadside in the freezing cold. It's two ladies who have come from a village and want to ask me in; they have so little but want to share it.

I'm learning a lot. Survival at –20 last year entailed taking any chance to bring my sleeping bags into the warm for a while if I reached a village. It's a mistake to do this at –40 or –50, because the amount of ice in the bags means that all is fine if the sleeping bags stay frozen as the interior of the bags is still very cosy, while the outside stays as a hard iced shell – and that's OK. If it starts melting then the water drips through and broaches the inner layers which then refreeze until I'm lying on icy surfaces at night when it all gets soggy

with my body-warmth. The bags get heavy with accumu-
lated ice, but I have to wait until there's a chance to thaw and
dry them thoroughly, a task that has to wait until I stop for
more than a day. The effects of my breathing are bad
enough. It's funny because I'll be sleeping head tucked deep
inside and be fine. As soon as I emerge from the depths in
the mornings, the vapour from breathing becomes ice, and
my eyelashes often get frozen shut and have to be rubbed
open to see – and my hats and balaclava become glued to my
ears. Any hair that escapes will be pure white with frost.

After 500km I arrive at Chita and am befriended by the
scientists of the Chita Institute of Natural Resources and
Ecology. Tatiana, Sveta and Natasha and their colleagues
hang every single item of my equipment up to dry and air,
even though this transforms their office into a jungle of
down and Gortex, complete with steaming puddles as they
turn up the radiators. Sveta invites me back to the flat where
she lives with her son and daughter, to sleep in a real bed.
But there's much more to having arrived here than just
being spoilt.

Like David against Goliath, this team of scientists has got
permission from the government to write a report recom-
mending the least environmentally damaging route for the
Chita section of the inevitable oil pipeline from Moscow to
Vadivostok. Tatiana explains that amidst the badlands and
swamps, and remains of Stalin's uranium mines, there exists
Chara Sands, a pure golden sandy desert, and the area also
has a precious wildlife habitat and forest. While my kit gets
sorted and dried, Tatiana and Natasha take me off on a two-
day field trip by air to the north Chita region to resurvey the

area before they write the report, in which they will advise against running it anywhere near Chara Sands. I feel privileged to be asked to go. It seems important. If you just travel through a land and don't give your support to causes within it that matter, you might as well just be watching it all on TV.

It's even more special than I expected. Digging through 10ft of snow at –50°C, Tatiana shows me the pristine golden sand dunes beneath all the ice, just like those in the Sahara. An even more vivid, enduring memory is Chara village, where we stay with Jakov and his family. Jakov was taken prisoner at 17 and survived working in mines as a driver, and building the road as a forced labourer on a diet of dried potatoes and 700gm of bread a day at –60°C. His imprisonment is long since over, but his exile from the Ukraine, his original home, is for ever. He married his wife Ludmila here, and their son Sasha goes to school at Chara.

Their house is simple, warm and friendly. They work hard to survive, attending to outside latrines and caring for their animals through fierce winters, like countless other Siberian households. But what gets to me is how he's grown to love the wild landscape that enslaved him and then gave him freedom to find ways to survive. He cares about the pipeline and the future of this environment. Bitterness isn't in Jakov's vocabulary. His mind isn't in the past. I'm only a layperson, but as an outsider and a British citizen I'm proud to be there and hope it just might help a bit. Above all, I feel I owe it to the the wilderness. I've lived in the open in the winter for months and the wilderness has looked after me. It's time to try to give something back. As always I receive more than I can give.

From the people in Chara, and when taking GPS and compass bearings with Tatiana in the woods, I've learned about the 'menu' in the forest that exists even in the dead of winter, with no berries, mushrooms or anything visible to sustain life. They've taught me the wilderness can be your own supermarket. Tatiana's tea recipe is as follows. 'Take coniferous branches, or twigs, put them in a teapot and boil. You can use the broth like a tea. Serve hot. Drink it. It tastes a bit like pine disinfectant, but it's full of vitamins.' Pine resin is also good for toothache. Aspen tree bark cures headaches. Best of all is birch tree bark, that tastes like British tea and can give all the vitamins your body needs.

On 22 February, I set off again, feeling the loss of leaving my friends.

Natasha writes in my journal:

Rosie, one more piece of advice. Very soon, you'll go through open spaces and steppe, without a forest. Spring will bring very strong winds. Stay in your tent, don't go when the wind is too strong. There are many roads in this world and I'm glad that your road and mine have crossed.

CHAPTER 23

A Siberian Bridge
Has No Middle

Siberia, March–September 2005

The riddle of Siberia is that nothing is as it seems. The fact that out of the white wilderness and the crystallised pine trees you can actually pick twigs and brew tea that has all the vitamins you require is just the start of it.

The enigma of this journey is that even in the middle of nowhere so much touches, moves, frightens me, gives me strength and makes me laugh too.

For example there are the wild dogs. I've been warned these packs of feral dogs have been known to attack people and are more dangerous than wolves, because they have no fear of man and are often starving. I'm on the first section of the really broken part of the road, with sharp rocks protruding through frozen quagmire. I'm having to do one kilometre at a time.

God said to love your enemies, I'm thinking, *but nobody could love this road.*

Suddenly I have the feeling I'm being watched. A large white dog appears out of nowhere in front of me and stands snarling.

'Go home!' I say in my best Russian.

Instead he comes closer, hackles raised, beautiful white ears flat back, barking and growling. A moment later about ten other wolf-like dogs arrive, encircling me and the cart. They came closer, baring their teeth in fury. They are emaciated, their ribs showing through their thick coats. Instinct takes over. On reflex I reach into the cart, get out my last loaf of frozen bread and throw it to them. One of the dogs catches it deftly in his jaws and runs off with it. The rest of them follow him – and that's that.

I don't go further than another 10km as the terrain is tiring. I park up for the night as usual, and go to sleep. I wake to find heavy lumps squashing the tent from outside. Then I hear a snoring sound.

I'm dreaming, I think. Shall I curl up in a ball and pretend it isn't happening or go out and investigate?

I open the flap very cautiously and take a peek. Stretched out sleeping all around me are seven of the dogs I encountered yesterday. They look completely at home. The big white dog raises his head, looking at me with his black eyes shining in the moonlight and starts wagging his tail. It's amazing what a little kindness can do. It seems they've decided to track and guard me through the night, in return for a bit of breakfast, before finally disappearing.

I run east from March to May, then turn north to Yakutsk. The landscape changes from dense forest to exposed tundra with high winds. When I camp at night I have to tie the tent to thick bunches of grass to hold it down, so the dome looks like a spider caught in the centre of a web. As the weather improves, I start meeting more people. Among the most interesting are scrap-metal collectors, who roam Siberia searching for remains of car and aeroplane crashes. One of them, Yuri, proclaims, 'We're very fashionable people. We're into recycling in a *big* way.' He's observed that one of Hercules's shafts is broken and kindly offers to mend it.

Then there's Valdimir, who approaches me in a cardboard-covered car to protect it against the highway's stones and shares his picnic, letting me listen to his Beatles album, his most treasured possession. Best of all is meeting Canadian explorer Colin Angus on a bicycle on his way to Moscow. He gives me a bar of chocolate; I give him my gritty coffee – not much of an exchange but at least I'm pleased I can lend him the antennae of my satphone to put a call through to his family, as his own is broken.

On 1 May, the Russian Easter, it's still snowing, and has become –25° with wind chill. But the ice floes on the River Lena have disappeared by the time I cross this frontier into Yakutia on a ferry. Within weeks, the weather changes from winter to a blazing cauldron. This region has one of the greatest extremes of temperature, ranging from –71.2° in winter and +40° in summer. It's become like the heart of Africa instead of Siberia. It's a surprise, even though I've known it's going to happen. The sky becomes so black with mosquito clouds that sometimes you'd think it was dark, even though beyond the swarms of bugs the sun is shining. It's endlessly sticky and the mosquitoes have a habit of making for one's mouth, ears and nose, and have soon bitten all the way down the inside of my throat. I get used to it and the warmth gives back time to do things: just using my hands without fear of freezing gives a whole new sense of freedom.

On 6 June at long last, after running for a year and eight months from Tenby, I reach Yakutsk N62 131E. Geoff flies out, bringing news of family and friends including my god-daughters at Kitezh. I hear that people are still sponsoring me to help Kitezh in a small but steady way. I'm overjoyed to see Geoff. It means more than anything because this is the last time until Magadan that I'll be in touch with home, except through brief satphone messages. The last chance too to get kit for the final 2450 miles in Russia. Geoff brings new shoes from Saucony and other valuable items, and also the present for Hercules of a little anti-rust paint, while Steve Holland sends new tyres for the wilderness ahead through DHL. The long arm of caring seems to reach me every-where and never stops.

I set off again along a lonely road, one of many tangents and dusty tracks leading east towards the river Aldan, when a car draws up with a beautiful dog in it. Four people get out and I say politely how much I admire the dog that remains bundled in the back of the car. His fluffy large frame and long tail fill the whole of the inside. He's like a big, tall fox, pure white. He's different from the wild white dogs, but seems to be one of the highly regarded Lika – a native Siber-ian hunting breed – looking like a valuable show dog.

The older people look grim. The young man with them, who may be their son, is almost in tears and suddenly blurts out, '*Podorak*! I have a present for you!' He's desperately trying to give me the dog. I explain, touched at his generos-ity but puzzled, 'I love dogs, but I can't have one right now because I'm on a long journey and can't look after him. Anyway, he's yours, he's so beautiful.' I explain that the hardest part of the run is ahead and I might not be able to feed him.

They drag the dog out, tail between its legs, head hanging down. There's a rope around its neck.

'Please take him,' the owner whispers in English. 'Please. My parents are taking him to the forest to shoot him.'

Without his parents noticing he's actually trying to cram a 100 rouble note into my hand to encourage me to take the dog. As I push the roubles back to him, I can see he loves this animal so much, he's trying to do anything to save him. I take the rope.

'His name is Dollar. He's eight years old. They're going to shoot him because he's eaten all their chickens,' he adds. 'He'll be good luck to you. Dollar means loads of bucks.'

Moments later they all leap into the car and sweep off, leaving me on the dusty road with the dog on a rope. Well, he has a better chance here than being shot.

I cut the rope and he runs free. He's the beautiful white shadow that follows me for ten days. He has such great times swimming in swamps, leaping through woods and bounding at full gallop to catch me up. Even on a diet of buckwheat, he thrives, gets fatter, and is full of gaiety and charm. We cross the Aldan River in a tiny boat borrowed off a villager, almost get shipwrecked, but arrive OK. This proves to be one of the easiest rivers as it's deep and navigable. Over the next 200km, life is easy. It's not so isolated yet and in this forested farming area we have all kinds of adventures.

The dog is very well behaved except when chasing chickens, cows or lorries, when he goes deaf. I spend my time training him, fleeing with him after he's got into a scrape with a farmer. But as he gets fatter, he stops chasing livestock altogether. Hunger made him do it, not vice. At last he can resist vehicles too, without going after them, and then I have to pat him and pet him for ten minutes, congratulating him for listening to me, so progress gets a bit slow. But he's learning and I'm learning too. Every midday he stops, lies beside Hercules and won't move for a while, which gets me into the siesta routine in the heat of the day, which is so wise. Then at night, once the tent is up, he's in it, on his back, waiting for his stomach to be stroked. He's the smartest dog I've ever known. When some drunken men pass close by at night, and I tell him to be silent, he doesn't give me away by barking. They pass on by without ever knowing we're there.

No person nor animal has shared my life on the road but I know it can't continue and worry about this all the time. In the remote areas ahead we'd starve; it would be very hard and dangerous and if the wild dogs returned they'd kill him, as would the wolves. They'd react very differently from when I was on my own. But food is my greatest concern. If I ran out of food, I'd suffer but I'd get through it, I hope. I can do that to myself, but not to an animal. If I put him through this and he survived, I wouldn't be able to take him out of Russia. I couldn't bear for Dollar to end up in a dog shelter, if such a thing exists in Magadan. He has to stay in his land, in the centre of Siberia, especially because Dollar only understands a limited amount of Russian. His main language it turns out, is Yakutian, the native tongue in this region.

I don't know how I can make a new life for this wonderful dog, but eventually, after ten days, I get to the small town
of Xanadu, where they still speak the Yakutian language. A
girl of about twelve puts her arms around Dollar, and her
mother starts petting him while he licks their faces, Their
expressions are full of caring and love for him. Dollar has
chosen his new home and his previous owner would have
been so happy. I give the girl the lead I've sewn for him out
of part of my old rucksack. I can tell they'll love him for ever
and he's been saved. They don't own chickens but I don't
think he'd chase them anyway if he had a good home, now
that I've trained him. But it breaks my heart. I give Dollar a
pat and hug, telling him to be good, and leave crying.

As I set off for Xanadu in early July I never imagine the next
1000 miles will take until September, yet this is what
happens.

The hardest part is crossing so many bridgeless rivers and
swamps. There are about forty rivers to cross, permanent
and temporary with many braids in just one section of about
270km. I'm often stuck: after crossing one river safely it
rains again and I have to camp by the banks and wait for the
rain to stop and the river-level to fall before fording the next
river. I measure the fall of the river with stones by the
water's edge inch by inch, praying it doesn't rain. Sometimes
it rains for days: the climate has changed again and it's
swamp and rainforest weather. I eke out food, looking for
berries and mushrooms, catching a few fish, using all the
natural nutrition the Institute taught me, and then some, a

plethora of pine-needle soup, rosehips, nettles, dandelions and blueberries, but I'm eternally anxious about running out of food. I keep an eye out for vehicles, but there are very few. When I can't afford to wait any longer I'll have to make a break for it. I don't trust my rope. So I try to get across with sticks and plan the safest route, and then make many journeys with the equipment bit by bit, wearing my shoes with neoprene socks, a great tip from Mark of Terra Nova Tents. I take Hercules empty last of all, bracing myself against the current pulling him downstream. It's very time-consuming. I'll never take bridges for granted again.

By 11 August I'm halfway through the maze of water and swamps. The next river doesn't look as dangerous as most. Heavy clouds overhead forecast a rainstorm and I have to get to the other side first. Right now the weather's calm and dry. I'm on my second journey across, this time pulling Hercules, when I suddenly slip. I hear the water roaring in my ears. I'm spluttering and coughing, clutching Hercules as we're swept downstream. A great log crashes into me, hitting me on the head. I feel my limbs being torn away by giant merciless hands, then everything goes black. Hercules has saved me while I'm unconscious. His red harness, with me still strapped into it, is clinging by the skin of its teeth to a sharp branch. I come to with a bursting headache, among a pile of logs buffeting each other and me. The log the harness caught is a half-sunken hunk.

My head is in agony but I'm safe and the flash flood has passed. I am completely disorientated and the rest of the night is a blur. With the help of the GPS I painfully retrace my steps, collecting all my belongings from the river banks.

The feeling of having been frightened and yet surviving is impossible to describe. Thank God I made it. They call this road built by Stalin's prisoners the Road of Bones, but I call it 'The Road of Courage'. One morning I look out of my tent at dawn to see a human skull and part of a skeleton unearthed by the floods. I'm devastated by pity and respect. The bones don't give a sense of horror, but of the triumph of a human spirit that survived even through death. I make simple crosses over the bones and say prayers for them.

There were around 300 concentration camps in this area alone. I shall never forget how the very few survivors I've met have a gentleness and kindness towards me as a stranger that overwhelms me in the face of the misery they've been through. Some of the Guardians of the Roadworks are very old men who've somehow lived through it all. Beyond Kiodene, I pass many deserted, abandoned villages that were the entrances to goldmines and part of the old concentration camp system. I finally reach the junction back to the main section of the Road of Bones, where rusting vehicles park together. A man climbs out of one, waving a vodka bottle, though he's not drunk. He's very elderly, painfully thin, and takes my arm and invites me into these vans linked together by treadways, that are apparently makeshift accommodations for Guardians of the Roadworks.

He shows me into the men's dormitory, beds covered with grey blankets, gesturing for me to lie down and rest. I do, just for a while. He takes off my shoes, tucking me in like a father. Later he wakes me up, taking me to another van that's 'the washroom'. He's heated water for me to wash in and produces a bar of soap and towel. He and two friends cook me dinner from the stores the construction company left for them. He shows me a faded photo of his wife and three children, now all dead. He's drunk a lot of vodka by the time dinner is served, but for me he gets out a bottle of pink non-alcoholic drink, because I'm a lady, he says. I've never felt so honoured, cared for or so moved.

The last river I have to cross is especially dangerous and flooded. I know it lies ahead, and have been worrying about it for a week. There have been no vehicles, nothing on the road, until I get within 15km of this river. An old truck on giant balloon wheels that can take on almost anything, draws up beside me like a blessing from God. It's like something out of John Bunyan. The family in the truck are on their way home to the province of Magadan. They say I must go with them or I won't get across this river.

The problem is I've nearly run out of food; the water is high and could remain so and there might not be any other help for weeks. Yet if I take the lift for this 15km and break my pledge to travel on foot except across water all the thousands of miles of run would have been for nothing. If your promise is broken then you are broken and strength is really gone. You can't fool yourself, but this delightful family understand – and have a solution. They say they'll take the cart ahead so I can run faster, then they'll simply wait by the river for me to arrive and still help me.

I set off quickly to avoid delaying them more than necessary. I leave them manhandling Hercules onto the truck. Shortly afterwards they pass me hooting and cheering me on as they go. A few miles later I realise that it's all happened so quickly and unexpectedly that I don't even have my passport or documents with me as they are in my bags in the cart. I don't even have any contact numbers and not a single rouble. Only trust. But I still can't help thinking, *What if there's been a misunderstanding?*

Of course they are there on the banks, waiting, cheering me again to the finish before the river, where they've prepared food and built a fire. Then Konstantin and Lena and their family bear Hercules and me across the raging torrent, setting me down on the other side. They understand all about my challenge and leave me to pull Hercules on from there. Next day, after the secondary road joins the big road going south and north, there they are again, searching for me, and they invite me to their village nearby. They ply me with home-grown tomatoes, berries and kindness and I have to prevent them giving me their only pair of sunglasses as a gift.

I meet Baglan on the main highway, ten days further on along the road to Magadan.

My notebook has somehow fallen off the cart and though I've retraced my steps I can't find it. I'm distraught, for it contains irreplaceable addresses and memories. A lorry stops and the driver, a tall, good-looking man, climbs down, shakes my hand and starts talking about a notebook. Thinking he wants to write in my notebook I sadly confess I've lost it. But he's trying to explain that he's *found* it by the roadside. He doesn't have it now, as he's travelling north on a long haul, but gives me his home address. He's taken it to Magadan and left it with his wife.

Only once in east Siberia do I have a difficult encounter and I suspect the person is not a true Siberian, because Siberian and Russian men are so very honourable to women. One morning, I hear a noise outside my tent and to my astonishment right outside is a man, completely naked except for the T-shirt he's wearing around his head like a balaclava, hiding his face. I only see his eyes peering out through the slits. He must be stark-raving mad because the mosquitoes gather around him in clouds as he waves a gun at me, speaking not a word – and he's playing with himself.

I can't just rush off and leave my kit and tent behind, especially not after keeping it together across all those rivers. The trick, I realise, is not to appear startled. That would unsettle him and rob him of my reaction. I'll always be quite proud that I manage to pack up everything, even retrieve every one of my valued fourteen tent pegs. I try to behave as if having a naked man outside with a gun is quite normal. I keep saying *niet* and *dasvadana*, and Hercules and I get away unscathed, but I dream of the troubled soul for many nights, and keep seeing faces in the trees.

After this I run headlong for Magadan. I'm on my 24th pair of shoes and have covered over 1500 miles in them. I pick pieces of car-tyre off the roadside and stick them on with Russian superglue I bought in the last village to give them a longer life. I put grass in the shoes for extra padding from the hard stones on the road as my feet are getting sore.

It's the countdown to Magadan at last. By the beginning of September, 120km ... 70km ... 50km ... *I'm coming to the finish of Russia after all that,* I think. *I've nearly got there.* 30km out of Magadan I sleep for the very last night under Siberian stars, overwhelmed by emotions of all kinds. I remember all those hundreds of nights in Siberian forests, beside rivers; the ghosts, the fear and fight to survive; and how I've somehow been looked after all the way through; about the honesty, courage and generosity of the Siberian people. It will never be the same. It's the end ... and a new beginning; a new continent ahead, people to love, a land to be discovered.

I find Baglan's home, a small top-floor apartment on the outskirts of Magadan. He's away driving the lorry, but his wife and daughter greet me with the torn blue bag that's fallen off the back of my cart, containing the precious note-book and my camera and purse. She won't take any reward, though life is tougher here economically than other parts of Russia: jobs are scarce, pensions are worth nothing. Life expectancy for men is 50 and going down. There's superficial glitz, fine shops, but the people here are forgotten by Moscow, so far away.

I arrive in Magadan in time to catch the last plane over the Bering Sea to Alaska before the winter. DHL Magadan takes charge of Hercules, and Lubya the manager shows me 'The Mask of Sorrow', the huge sculpture standing above Magadan as a monument to the gulag prisoners.

'Magadan has the longest high street in the world,' Lubya says, 'because it's part of the 1000 miles of the Road of Bones. The fact that misery, pain and death marked the foundation of Magadan doesn't mean it has ended its history in this way. Hard times now can end with faith and work. One day Magadan will be a beautiful and prosperous place.'

Next day, DHL take me to the airport, delivering me with the same care as if I were one of their parcels. They hug and kiss me and are the last people I see in Siberia. I can hardly bear to speak. As I look back at Magadan out of the plane window and think forward to the wild, beautiful country that lies ahead, I feel that too many of my prayers have already been granted for just one lifetime.

On 17 September, I touch down in Alaska.

CHAPTER 24

Falling in Love
with Alaska

Alaska, September–October 2005

To arrive in the dark, at 4am, in a new continent after a year
and a half in Russia, is a feeling I can hardly describe. I am
overwhelmed as I walk out of the airport. Everything is
entirely different. The smell of the mountain air, the vibrant
atmosphere and feeling of life.

I see the outline of the snow-covered Chugach Mountains
behind the city of Anchorage emerging at dawn and am also
struck by the loneliness of Alaska. Away from the city, my
journey here is going to be harder than Siberia.

I book in at a campsite near the town centre where the
leaves are already falling from the trees like golden coins. It
feels extraordinary to be speaking in English for the first
time since the UK. On my first day in Anchorage, everybody
seems to be stopping to say, 'Hi, have a *good day!*' After all
these months in the frozen wilderness the ordinary bustle of
life feels magical. I am entranced by the tall, modern buildings, busy streets, lively cafes, well-stocked food stores and
forests of T-shirts in the clothes shops.

While I wait for Hercules to arrive from Magadan,
Anchorage becomes the vital staging post for the next part

of my run. My plan – and dream – is to set off from the westernmost tip of the North American continent, from a village on the Bering Strait astonishingly and aptly called Wales. Though –60°C in Siberia, at least I am mostly on a road. Over 1000 miles of my route in Alaska will be across bogs, marsh, mountains, long stretches of frozen waterways and sea-ice. I have to be sure I get the correct information regarding the route, for my equipment to be as precise as possible. Although I am longing to get going I have to wait for vital equipment and make sure I am totally prepared for this very dangerous section of my run. It would be irresponsible to leave until I am as safe as I can make myself for the challenge. As I set off every day on quests for Geological Survey maps, electronic maps to be loaded on my GPS, repairs and kit organised by the camping store REI, I receive discounts and favours and kind remarks: 'Stay safe,' 'Praying for you,' 'Go for it gal,' even 'Will you marry me?'

I'm inspired and awed by the help I receive over the next few months. Just as in Russia, people's actions and generosity make all the difference to whether I'll make it or not.

My campsite neighbours are unforgettable.

I had been told that the campsite, though well appointed with pretty trees, isn't in a good area of town, and many people living here drink a lot, but they've all read about me in the papers and seem to take pride in every small step I make in my preparations. In the tent field there are some people who have nowhere else to sleep and many problems. Yet they're totally honest regarding my possessions and all look out for me.

Freddie, who cares for his sick brother Larry, says he'll 'eyeball' any stranger who comes to my tent. Another man (who like me is on the run, though in his case from someone who wants to kill him) is obsessed with *Jane Eyre* and lends me books. Then Mark weaves his way unsteadily over to my tent, saying he's concerned for my sake about the bears in the wilderness. *'I gotta teach you how to shoot!'* His eyes close and he collapses asleep outside my tent until his girlfriend drags him back to theirs. John doesn't drink at all and has a brown dog Buster who rushes out in haste on his long lead at night for a pee and runs around the tent, tying his master up in knots inside.

When it's my birthday, the campers come over at 3am inviting me to a party. I'm very touched but I'm sleepy and politely decline. They're back again at 7am and leave a note. I'm already in town phoning my family. When I return, nobody talks to me, nobody comes over. I think, I'm only here for a few more days, so I'm sorry if I've offended them. They don't let me near their tents when I try to apologise. Then suddenly, all is revealed. They come with a birthday cake, ordered and somehow paid for. It's beautiful, expertly iced, with ROSIE written on it – and there's a little pink heart on it too. They give me a white T-shirt, which they've all signed.

Freddie says, 'You give me hope.'

I've contacted the Iditarod Sled Dog Race Committee. Much of my route will be along the course of the legendary Iditarod covering 1200 miles of wilderness from Anchorage to Nome every March. My route from Wales, Alaska will hopefully end in Nome. From there I can follow the Iditarod route in reverse to Anchorage or, weather not permitting this, to Fairbanks.

The organisers have been extremely helpful, putting me in touch with Carolyn Craig and Will Peterson, who for years have been among the dedicated Volunteer Sweep Team for the Race. Will and Carolyn mix enthusiasm with a sense of reality and their ability to reach beyond the odds – maybe to do with the spirit of the Iditarod – and find ways to get there. Some people you can describe by how they look, others by the feelings coming from them. The way they help me is exceptional. The problems and uncertainties of my journey are very real, but they trust me to do my best and give me wonderful support.

The Iditarod is more of a navigational route than a trail in the exact sense and much of it is open rivers and swamps. If I could wait until March the great rivers, sea bays, marsh, mountains and swamps would be frozen and packed down by snowmobiles to make a safer path. I can't wait that long and need to risk crossing it now. I still have so far to go. I know it will be treacherous and half frozen, but Carolyn and Will's information and advice may make it possible.

'We have a network of friends all along the trails,' Carolyn says, 'and we'll keep track of you.' Will writes a detailed trail guide for me, with phone numbers and contacts in all the off-road villages along the Iditarod route, and inserts waypoints on my GPS showing the wilderness shelters and the especially dangerous areas between Nome and Anchorage.

The DHL Office becomes the meeting of east and west. On 4 October, Hercules arrives in triumph from Russia, and it feels like being reunited with an old friend, while Geoff, those at Saucony, PHD and others send parcels from the UK, including the mended and cleaned extreme-weather sleeping bags and the mighty PHD Mustagh down jacket. My third winter on the run is coming. I can't believe it.

Next day, Carolyn comes dancing down to the campsite with tremendous news. 'It's all going even better than I could ever have thought,' she says. Her friend, Dr Adrian Ryan, has phoned her. Dr Ryan, an orthopaedic surgeon and native Alaskan from Unalakleet, halfway to Wales, says he'll be flying to Unalakleet in his Piper Navajo in a few days to visit his mum. Do Rosie and Hercules want to come? One of the big problems is getting to the Bering Strait for the start of the run. Carolyn has been looking for a way to get me there. My journey truly has guardian angels.

I say farewell to my campsite friends and for the last few days of frantic preparation move to the home of Carolyn's sister Shannon and husband Charlie Bader, who've also become great allies along with their mum Ella. While packing, a Japanese radio station keeps calling, asking for an interview with 'Miss Rosie'. It all comes together amazingly. Charlie has always planned to overhaul Hercules but there's very little time. He does what he can, brilliantly patching the big holes the Siberian logs and stones tore in Hercules, and painting him with epoxy resin. Will puts a sticker on Hercules's backside saying ALASKA GIRLS KICK ASS! as a finishing touch. Then we're ready to go.

*   *   *

Friday, 7 October dawns beautiful and clear, the first frost sparkling on the grass and fallen leaves, as Hercules is loaded up to go the airport.

As a finale, Charlie makes a video for my family. 'Where are you from?' he asks, as I speak into the camera.

'Wales.'

'And where are you going now?'

'*Wales!*'

The little plane with Adrian flying and his son Jonathan as co-pilot flies high over the Alaska Range then dips down to view the endless terrain. The vast, blinding, mesmerising wilderness, mountains, valleys, rivers, forests shun you and call you, climbing into your mind and soul, just to look down on them. I can see so much at once, that's how in one way it's different from Siberia, where I've never had a bird's eye view. But also, as I look down on it all, there's a sense of freedom as well as struggle here, not the pain, not the prison camps, so very different from Siberia even though so close geographically.

Right now, whatever lies in front of me, I feel that something will happen to me in this land that will for ever change the way I think about life. Even while thinking, *How shall I do it, how shall I really cross it on foot?* I know the price won't be too high, because no price can be. At this moment I fall in love with Alaska.

We touch down at little Unalakleet airport at sunset; crimson and scarlet light spreads in exquisite beauty over Norton Sound and the Bering Sea.

Eva, Adrian's mother, is small, slight, bounding with energy. There are lots of family and children around, warmth from the heart and warmth from the fire. There is traditional food on the table: moose stew, salmon caught in the summer and smoked, home-made bread and cookies. Also Chinese noodles from the little store in town because the children like them so much.

Adrian's sister, Ferno Tweto, a perky, attractive, fit-looking lady with short hair and a mischievous twinkle, is a renowned runner. 'Women like you and me are completely crazy,' she assures me. Everyone is full of jokes and good humour. Overcome with it all and sleepy, I'm soon tucked in bed under a satin-covered feather quilt in a pretty room.

I shall be running through Unalakleet on my way down the Bering Strait, so I leave some of the maps and other kit I don't need immediately. Next morning, Adrian and Jonathan fly me on to Wales – 224 air miles further north. Adrian won't take any money for this expensive, complicated flight.

The wind is gusting to 30mph as we land on the airstrip in Wales. The plane shudders in the wind on the runway as Hercules and I hastily disembark. Adrian gives me his pilot's gloves as a talisman, and for warmth and luck. Moments later they have taken off. I wave until they are a speck high over Cape Prince of Wales. To seaward clearly visible are Little Diomede Island, part of the US, with Big Diomede behind it, which belongs to Russia. Just two miles separate them. In between is the International Date Line and USA/Russian border. So Big Diomede is only 30 miles from Wales; East Cape in Siberia 55 miles. So close.

Black clouds hang over the islands. The light of an icy gleam of sunshine from somewhere shines up beneath these clouds, illuminating their outline. I think, *I'll go back to Siberia one day across the Bering Strait. No ice bridge now*. But I vow that when my run is done, I'll get sponsorship, and like the Asiatic tribes and one or two intrepid modern travellers these days, attempt this expedition next. I wouldn't have given up the Road of Bones for anything, but there always has to be an unfinished dream in a person's heart; the hunger of reaching forwards to next time.

The wild beach stretches out towards flat land, but behind me in the lee of the rocks are the cluster of buildings that is Wales Village, home to 152 inhabitants, the westernmost inhabited 'city' on the continent of North America.

I walk from the airstrip down the only street in the village, along which are low-lying little homes, a small white church and Kingiknuit School. Adrian told me it has just 48 pupils to 12th grade. I don't think I was expected, but people may have heard something about it on their handheld, radios, Internet – or the bush telegraph! A lady rushes towards me in an ATV off-road buggy, like a golf cart, an integral part of modern life in Wales, with several children clinging on precariously. Lena is ebullient, with dark-brown eyes, the only part of her face visible, as she's wearing a big hat and several scarves. People suddenly appear from nowhere, crowding around me, maybe most of the population. Lena and Marie and several other kind people ask me to stay. Unable to choose, and because it's what I want most dearly to do, I explain I'd love to sleep by the shore, because I've always wanted to look out on Diomede Islands. They invite me to put up the tent up anywhere I wish. I camp on the wild beach. The wind is still howling, but the tent is sheltered behind a sand dune. I wake in the night, listen to the crashing waves, giving thanks for being able to have made it here, then go to sleep again amid the sweet smell of the tundra and mosses beneath the slight covering of snow. At this time of year the really cold weather has not yet set in and it's only −10°C.

All except two of the population are Inuquik Eskimos. It's a tough place to live. No vegetables will grow, no trees. Hunting and fishing are the only food source except for supplies flown in, and everything is very expensive. I learn from the villagers that the wind never stops. On Christmas Day last year a man left his home during a gale to walk just 100 yards to another house in the village and was blown out to sea, his body never discovered. Yet life is organised in resourceful ways. There's a small health clinic, even a launderette, managed in winter with snow-water melted by the electric plant; electricity from a wind turbine station; a community centre and small shop. Much is closed as tomorrow is Sunday and on Monday it's Columbus Day. I'm shown over Kingikmuit School; the students sign my Red Dragon Flag and draw pictures of Hercules and me to inspire me. A teacher takes photos, sending them through the school's internet to James so that Wales, UK can immediately enjoy them. Pastor Matt says prayers for me in church and, as an extra precaution, lends me a Smith & Wesson pistol to frighten off bears. Then, the next day on 12 October I set off to find my way across the York Mountains to Brevig Mission.

* * *

As Carolyn and Will warned, it's a hard time of year. From Wales I have to proceed to Brevig and then to Teller and Nome, where I'll pick up the Iditarod Route. To get to Brevig from Wales, apart from air travel, normally means going by boat or snowmobile on sea-ice, which would have been good for me but the sea hasn't yet frozen. That is why I have to go over the York mountains via the Kandugak valley. After the first few miles beyond Tin City Radar Station the foreshore ends, the mountains dropping sheer to the sea, so this inland route is the only way. It does exist, the villagers say, but it's difficult and rarely if ever used.

The actual distance from Wales to Brevig is only 60 miles. I have estimated that it will take me 7–8 days to get there but instead it takes 16. Any hopes that Alaska might be any easier than Siberia vanish. It's a beautiful journey but a struggle.

The first stretch is simple: an 11-mile rough road leads to Tin City US Radar Station. The radio operators spoil me. I have a shower, a delicious meal, and then set off again as it's only early afternoon. I proceed along the foreshore as there are no more trails after Tin City, and later camp among the driftwood and mounds of soft snow, watching a giant orange fairy-tale moon rise up and balance on snowy hills.

Next morning, before going much further, a voice behind me shouts, '*Hi, this is meals on wheels!*' An ATV buggy rears over the dunes. It's Ben, one of the Tin City radio operators, bearing army iron rations. Lena and Larry from Wales arrive with a jar of seal oil and a snack of home-cured salmon sticks, wanting to check on me before I head into the wilderness of mountains and valleys beyond the range of their ATVs. They assure me they'll be waiting for satphone messages. 'Remember, this is Alaska. We'll get help to you if you need it.' Alaskans always do what they can for you.

I don't see another person for ten days. I haul Hercules over the brow of the first hill, away from the sea and descend into endless valleys, with countless wilderness rivers to cross, mostly by wading and making my way through the ice, which is not yet thick. The water is cold even though not yet fully frozen. As in Russia, I wear neophrene diving socks to protect me. In this way at least it is one world: the same equipment works.

The mountains rise steeply either side. There is ice with over-falls up to my knees in the Kandugak River Valley, with areas of sharp boulders in between so it's slow going. I can hardly move with the wheels on, and not without them either as Hercules' bottom is getting wrecked again and here it is harder to pull him as a sled. I have to keep taking the wheels on and off with frozen fingers. It takes a lot of concentration not only to avoid losing the hubs caps, but to put the wheels on straight afterwards. If I don't the bearings will be damaged. As I climb up again, making towards a pass I have to get through, I enter a world of pure snow and ice, with majestic mountains soaring either side, a world that makes me feel very small and humble. I've only seen two grizzly bears on the tundra and they're as wary of me as I am of them. I haven't had to try out the noise of the Pastor's gun. Now there are just magnificent bald eagles wheeling high above the mountains, watching me, on wonderful wings I wish I had. I love gazing at them. I find it hard to take it in that I am completely alone in this rare and beautiful place. It's definitely worth the struggle.

There are so many creeks. The third turn on the left leads to Rapid Creek and I mustn't miss it. There's just whiteness and washed outlines of the mountains as it starts snowing. *Don't stay on the same compass course too long*, I think. *Don't miss the turning*. I follow the GPS trail-lines, but the maps are old. There are precipices and giant chunks of ice like fallen icebergs broken off from the mountain ledge across the GPS trail-line. Like desert sands the snow wilderness constantly changes, hiding its past. My progress is slow but the GPS keeps me going in the right direction.

Suddenly the weather closes in and I have to hole up in the tent for two days to wait it out. The storm winds and blizzards are relentless but the tent is grand. It's a pedigree mountain tent. I put a call through on the satphone to Wales and to Tin City to tell them I'm absolutely well but will be overdue at Brevig. I use the time to rest, look after myself and keep planning every step ahead on the maps. At this stage every ounce of weight counts – I am not carrying a book, an iPod or anything like that. It's tough enough just to keep the GPS in batteries and carry the heavy Solar charger. I rig up during brief respites in the weather to give emergency power to the satphone.

The weather eventually clears but it's a very steep climb to the pass. I have to unload Hercules, just like when I was crossing the rivers, and carry the bags ahead, which takes all my energy.

I feel fantastic when I finally make over the highest pass on 24 October and begin descending to Lost River. I can see the sea and coast again. The terrain turns into tundra, bog and beaches and seems easier than the mountains, but there are many half-frozen creeks. Most of the creeks have a strong ledge of ice for a few feet from either bank and rushing water in the middle.

The only way to get across them is to slither along the ice as it is too tough to break and drag the sled with me. Going on all-fours works best as I'm steadier – huskies know a thing or two. I fling a cloth or rug ahead of me to make a grip for my knees but in the end the cart always falls into the water in the middle of the creek and I have to haul it out the other side. It's exhausting and takes ages. Hercules, who weighs about 200lb with all the kit doesn't float any more – maybe there's too much ice, and he's getting old.

I start running out of food before the end of this stretch despite iron rations, as the weather has delayed me. Fortunately I have heaps of purely natural vitamins of very high quality, sent to me by Brian Welsby and part of the regime for his Olympic athletes. I cook the vitamins with water to make soup and keep drinking this brew with seal oil, tasting of cod liver oil with attitude. This is powerful stuff, and very good for you. I find another Eskimo gift tucked away: a tiny bag with lumps of walrus blubber, which goes down well. The fat stops me from feeling too hungry even though I am not really eating enough calories.

The big fear always when you're alone is that you might lose it, like many a marathon runner who tries too hard. I simply cannot afford to let this happen as I am completely alone. One of the tent poles breaks during a gale in a fairly exposed part of the foreshore. It's a long night with the tent just wrapped around me. I shiver and shake. I can't fix it until the weather eases off next morning. Meanwhile, before the weather calms down enough for me to be able to fix it next morning, I set off early into the gale as the effort will warm me up. The danger is that if one thing goes wrong, it will have a domino effect. Perhaps it's because I am so cold when I set off that it happens. All of a sudden I miss my footing and fall hard on my ribs. I feel a searing pain and think I must have broken one. I wrap a scarf around my ribs and the pain becomes bearable. Maybe it is only cracked. I keep telling myself that I am strong from pulling the heavy cart. My muscles are good, and this helps keep the rib in place. I am absolutely determined to pull Hercules to Brevig now that I am so close. I have to grit my teeth a bit, but it's true what all the wise people say – if it's important enough, it is possible to keep going no matter what. I adjust the harness straps to go around my waist instead of my sides to make it less uncomfortable. It only takes two days to get to Brevig and by the 27th I've become much too full of excitement and adrenalin to feel any discomfort at all because I'm *only three miles from the end of this stretch!* It has been a special journey. I've been slow but I *have* stayed safe.

It's a wonderful clear day. I carry on back to the shore after taking a boggy inner route along Brevig Lagoon. I'm looking out for the first sight of the village, for a gap in the dunes and for people. The eagles are high in the sky. I pass a big herd of shaggy musk ox taking their ease in the chilly sunshine and peering at me over the dunes from the tundra behind.

Suddenly I see an old man and a little boy on the beach ahead of me. The first people I've seen for ten days. He introduces himself with a solemn handshake. Henry Olanna, collecting driftwood for the fire with his nephew. He has a look of disbelief on his face. He offers me a ride into town on his ATV which I refuse with thanks, because it's only one mile. I'm mad with joy at getting here. Henry returns as I reach the village.

'My wife says I gotta take you *home!*'

CHAPTER 25

There's No Place Like Nome

Alaska, November 2005

'I'm so thankful you got here!' says a villager, rushing over to me. 'The last woman to make it alone on foot through the Kandugak valley was Mrs Tocktoo running away from her husband in 1916.'

The wind has picked up again and is now screaming; black clouds hang low over the little tin houses, with walkways and a rickety bridge; the sagging wire from the fragile electricity system; a post office that's just a red metal box. There's ice, snow and swamps. Like Wales, Brevig is a place to which no roads lead and there are hardly any vehicles. There's no point, just snowmobiles, ATVs, a school, church, and so on. Life is pretty basic.

I'm knocked out that apparently people here amidst their own difficult existence have followed my progress in the mountains through the brief satphone calls I've made to Wales and Tin City, which have been passed on to them.

I'm planning to camp, but Rita Olanna throws her arms around me, drawing me into the house. 'We were beginning to worry about you during the storms,' she says. 'Even though you said you were fine, if you hadn't got here in two more days, Henry was going to go out and find you. Now we believe you can survive any sort of weather.'

My image of the evening is of warmth and kindness as a powerful entity; my sleeping bags and clothes being dried beside the wood stove; and a generous, nourishing meal. Native Alaskan people here as in Wales are subsistence hunters and fishermen and have been for generations. There's a shop, but it's limited, Rita explains. We dine on cornbread, walrus blubber, moose stew and seal oil, and cranberries picked from the tundra during the summer and pickled. Afterwards, they give me painkillers for the rib and a nice soft bed to sleep in. I find it harder to get out of this bed than to burrow up from my sleeping bag and tent when completely buried in snow.

Next morning I feel much better. I'm determined to get going again as soon as possible. The 90-mile stretch to Nome is partly a wilderness road. It's already closed for the winter due to extremely perilous weather conditions but locals say it's do-able, and won't be as hard as the run from Wales to Brevig. The toughest stage of wilderness is after Nome. I need to get the final preparation and logistics sorted in Nome; and my head is already there. I visit the clinic where the nurse says the rib is broken but not in a dangerous place. I call Carolyn in Anchorage after buying a phonecard, purchase dried fish from Henry, and spaghetti and coffee from the little store; and visited Pastor Crockett to return the Pastor in Wales's gun as promised. Pastor Brian Crockett has a team of husky dogs, and lends me one, a retired little old lady aged 10 called Sandy, with tawny fur, soft ears and gentle eyes for a day or so. I'll pull Hercules myself, but have Sandy to guide me over the difficult terrain. She'll pick her way through the ice on the shore to prevent me falling again.

I say goodbye to Rita and Henry and all the friends I've collected here; and also to Henry's dogs – for he has a dog team too, with a beautiful grey lead dog called Diesel who's the pride of his life. The dogs live outside, but have access to individual wooden kennels with cosy soft straw in them.

'Hey, Henry loves those huskies better than he loves me,' Rita jokes.

I set off for six miles along a thin strip of beach to the Nook and Imuruk Basin Outlet to the Bering Sea. The Imuruk Outlet is a roaring wild seaway 500 yards wide with deep, tossing water. Between Nook and Teller on the other side there's no way across except by boat, until it's frozen. I've been told to wait here until a fishing boat appears, hail it and pay them to take me across. Soon some Eskimo seal hunters come chugging into view from seaward, in a battered old tin boat they're deftly handling in fierce currents. They've been out fishing and hunting for two days though without much success they say. At the helm is an old man with a faraway seafaring look in his eyes, like a Native Alaskan Ancient Mariner. There's a young boy as crew who has no difficulty in balancing Hercules and dog and me somehow on board. It's fun.

The road is wild. No telegraph poles, fences, crossroads, just raw wilderness, windswept open tundra. I only have Sandy for two days. Once I'm on the road, the terrain is very harsh on her paws. She's old and not in training. Even though I like her company, and she is sweet and good-natured, I'm worried about getting Sandy home before I've gone too far. We're lucky because after two days of bad weather the first tough four-wheeled vehicle that bursts through the blizzards has in it good friends of Joe Garnie, the legendary husky musher who I had met in Teller, and who is also a friend of Brian's. So Sandy is taken to Joe's and then by him on to Brevig. I call the Pastor on the satphone later to check she's got home, and learn she is happy and eating well.

It takes nine days to reach Nome. Mostly I'm extremely lonely, but any vehicle that does pass brings a new story, like the day I meet the Mayor of Teller. Among Alaska's finest traditions are the wilderness shelters, kept unlocked for travellers. There's always food, matches and candles left there. Everyone who arrives can use what they need. The custom is to leave firewood chopped and food and anything else you don't require that might be useful to the next person. I stop in one of the two shelter cabins on my route one night. It's cosy but has been left a bit untidy, so I remove a bag of garbage which might attract rodents, hauling it onto Hercules. But what to do with it next is a problem. I'm still a long way from Nome. Fate is on my side though: the first car for two days zooms into view soon after I set off, and stops.

'Please could you take my rubbish for me?' I ask the smiling driver, explaining what I'm doing, and that I can't haul it to Nome.

'My pleasure!' he exclaims, leaping out of the car and almost bowing. 'I'm Ken Hughes, the Mayor of Teller. I always take the garbage.'

Among other splendid people are the TelAlaska Engineers, out in all weathers: they have to climb telephone towers and repair the system even at –40 or –50. Most of them, like Andy, are in fact mountaineers. Andy and his boss Roger say I can stay in the TelAlaska Hospitality house when I reach Nome.

On 5 November, I'm feeling rough. My rib's hurting again and I've only managed six miles a day for the last couple of days. A short time earlier there's been a white-out, with below zero temperatures, and blowing snow again. I'm pulling Hercules up a steep hill when a vehicle draws up. Inside are two charming men, the driver, John Earthman, and his passenger, Bob Collins, and a beautiful large falcon which they've been out flying. They ask if I'm all right. I give them a résumé of what I'm doing. After a while John asks me to join them for dinner which his wife is organising at their home 20 miles further on near Snake River on my route.

'I accept in spirit,' I say, 'and it's very kind of you to ask, but I don't think I'll make it in time.'

Imagine being invited to dinner in the middle of a white-out on a wilderness road. Bob later described how on the way out they'd seen something in the willows and thought they had a moose in their sights, before realising it was someone camping. Later after the blizzard descended and they decided to return to town, they'd seen me proceeding with Hercules.

'Maybe it's another crazy person pulling a bathtub for a "challenge",' John said. Because I had on big clothes and am tall, they didn't know if I was a man or a woman until they talked to me. Then they didn't know what I looked like, my age or anything as only a few inches of my face were visible from under the balaclava and my big hood.

After talking to them I feel better, and decide to accept their invitation after all – and actually make it in time for dinner, after pulling Hercules through more of the deep drifts on the road. When I finally arrive, John's wife Marguerite is so kind, and takes my wet clothes off to dry them. I have a wash and eat a pizza with them. It's great to be with his family and Bob and their friends, Dave and Seeni Holly. John and Bob are master falconers who live for the wilderness and know so much about it. The Peregrine Fund/World Centre for Birds of Prey in Boise, Idaho, has saved the peregrine falcon and many other species including the Mauritius kestrel and California condor, from extinction. Falconry is all about conservation and respect for the environment. Among the big problems for wildlife every-where are habitat and the spraying of chemicals in third world countries, with widespread effect on birds.

Bob gets ready to leave, saying, 'I must go to look after my girls.' He means his three setter dogs. 'They keep me busy.'

As he lives in Nome, he says I should call him if I need anything. It's a great privilege to be helped by this exceptional man. His father died from prostate cancer and that prompted him to become 'volunteer Alaskan HQ' of my run. Through his smart thinking and generosity he saves my life not just once but many times. Though he wouldn't think of it like that – he'd just say, 'There she goes again.'

The following morning I finally run into Nome. It's a beautiful sparkling Sunday; although cold, about −20, it's lovely and bright. As I come in from the north I see a clutch of buildings, the spire of a church, wild sea and the snow- and ice-covered landscape behind. It's so strange and uncanny. I'm arriving at the first town in the North Ameri- can continent. A town completely unconnected to any other by a road system, the oldest town in Alaska. A sign says 'WELCOME TO NOME, EST 1901'. In 1898 'Three Lucky Swedes' discovered gold in nearby Anvil Creek. Quickly 20,000 came to prospect for gold. Nowadays Nome has a population of about 4000 but still looks like a frontier town. I run along Front Street past the Board of Trade Saloon, oldest in Alaska, and the Nome Nugget newspaper office to reach TelAlaska House near the other end of town.

During the next eight days everyone pulls out the stops helping me. Hercules is put in the heated garage, Chuck Titus, Andy Hennings and the other TeleAlaskans repair and modify him, even paint on the name HERCULES. Chuck, who teaches the scouts wilderness survival, lends me his goggles, mitts and cleats; Operations Manager Roger Meeks offers an invaluable survival suit, Mayday device, strobe- light, and much more.

Bob comes over next day, driving me to town to search for thick waterproof storm trousers to use with my down trousers. It's soon going to be *very cold*. He helps greatly getting food, maps and discussing equipment. I've asked Geoff to get me another bivvi bag from Terra Nova. It's a nice strong red bivvi, and arrives safely. It's difficult to decide whether to bring the bivvi, which is lighter, or the tent which is more comfortable; because the load is extremely heavy, and I have to bring extra food, batteries

and stores, as ahead of me is arguably one of the toughest
stretches of the entire world run There are many questions
about maps, logistics gear and how much assistance I may
get from the remote roadless Eskimo villages, etc. to discuss
with everybody.

The State Troopers in Nome have been very helpful. I
listen carefully to their advice, which is to be vigilant. They
say that, as I know, winter wilderness conditions are life-
threatening. Every year people in this area die yards from
homes in the extreme weather. I'm passionately determined
to stay as safe as I can on the trail. There's a lot to organize.
The very charming Dr Lew at Norton Sound Regional
Hospital gives me a medical check and tells me my health is
first class. My only problem, she proclaims with a wry smile,
is that I have half of Siberia in my ears, and it's a wonder I
can hear at all. She spends nearly an hour syringing them
until my ears feel like roaring waterfalls.

I also get caught up in a whirlwind of interest in my journey. The day I arrived in Nome, journalist Marijke Engel
and photographer Jorg Modow flew in from Germany to
cover my run for *Brigitte* magazine. Marijke has contacted
me through the website. A Japanese radio station is trying to
get hold of me and thanks to James there have been thousands of hits on the web site. It's totally unexpected. I'm
about to charge off into the wilderness and James says,
'People are holding their breath to see what's going on.' I'm
amazed there's so much interest and it suddenly hits me that
this run is no longer just about me.

Nome made dreams come true during the Gold Rush and
so it's apt that another dream had become real here. Marijke

struggled for two years to get a commission to write about my journey, and has obtained one at last to get here with the amiable Jorg. They are pretty special people and just fit in and become part of the 'Nome A Team'. They even borrow my tent and come camping with me in the bitter cold, while I'm testing the bivvi. On their final evening she makes supper at TelAlaska House to say thank you to everybody, serving delicious pumpkin soup. Nobody, in the absence of many fresh vegetables, can understand how she got the ingredients.

Finally everything is ready and, after saying goodbye to friends I'll never forget, I set off from Nome. The Eskimos of the Alaskan coast, seeing me with my gear, ask sympathetically whether I'm on the run from the police.

'Not yet,' I reply. 'The State Troopers have all been wonderful. I'm on the run for another reason.'

CHAPTER 26

Surviving in Alaska

Alaska, November 2005

Hello James. Your mother left Nome midday yesterday, 14th November, on her way to White Mountain along the Iditarod trail. Last night and this morning the weather was about −30C with wind chill. She's walking along the coast of the Bering Sea with almost no natural shelter from the wind in many places. She asked me to paraphrase her thoughts for you as she enters this upcoming stage of her journey. She needs to keep absolute focus. Small mistakes have serious ramifications. She's more prepared now than ever for another arctic winter. Hercules has been further modified thanks to the kind folks at TelAlaska. She has a survival kit and an emergency May Day beacon. She wanted to say thank you to everybody and expresses her love for her family. She apologises for not having been in contact with all of you as much as she would like. She needed her time in Nome to prepare for the very difficult next stage. She remains committed to her family and friends and the causes in which she believes.

Bob Collins

The next months are the hardest of my run. There's never a time I feel like giving up, but many times I can't move forward and think I can't survive; when I'm so cold I'm afraid to sleep in case I never wake up, and nearly starve. Yet the danger is overshadowed by the logistical efforts of those who keep on supporting me. I dedicate these following chapters to you. I've never known such caring and it's true: love conquers all adversity.

From the start I sense there's more about this than just the hard physical journey and deadly cold. My images on the road along the shore from Nome are of beached fishing boats, roaring wind, driftwood sticking up from the snow like mooses' antlers; of passing a sign saying 'TRAVEL BEYOND THIS POINT NOT RECOMMENDED' and of Millie (wife of TelAlaska engineer Andy Hennings) driving through a five-foot snowdrift on the road to hand me a thermos mug of hot chocolate and give me a hug.

Three days later after very slow progress I'm still on my first 22km on an open strip of land between the stormy, icy expanse of the Safety Sound and the Bering Sea; the wind crashes over the road from empty spaces either side, as if riding its own freeway. Often I can't stand up in the gusts. I'm sheltering among driftwood in the bivvi when Bob appears after forcing his vehicle with huge care along the road. It's wonderful to see him. In spite of paparazzi there's absolutely no record of the hard parts of my run and he's determined to make a video for my family.

It's −32°C this morning. I don't know how he can even hold the camera – it's torture just to open the bivvi flap, as the snow packs the inside in moments. There must be more blobs than picture in the lens. Not much point in worrying 'what's my best profile' anyway as an inch of face is all that's visible. But thankfully the storm gusts ('blowholes') stop as suddenly as they start, and he can take wild but *slightly* calmer pictures, filming me running on the road to the Safety Roadhouse, a landmark closed and boarded up but which gives some shelter outside its walls. He sends the film to ITV News Wales so folks in Tenby can see it. I don't know how his hands hold out doing the photography. He just smiles encouragingly, saying 'Nose to the lens, that's pretty,' as if I were a film-star. Stuff like this helps my morale more than anything else on earth.

I'm stuck for three days outside the Safety Roadhouse by the weather. It is difficult enduring the cramped conditions in the bivvi in deep ice and snow and the wind is too strong to risk emerging. It would be far too dangerous to attempt walking into the wind. It's −30 and twice as cold as it was during my first year near Riga, when I lived in the bivvi at about −20. Now it's too cold to even open the flap and it's like being in a body-bag covered in ice and snow. The bivvi may be light and low-lying but I dream of my tent and am so glad it's being repaired and sent to Unalakleet, 280 miles ahead.

On 19 November the wind eases and I set off resolutely over the Safety Bridge, thinking, *This is my very last bit of road for the next 1000 miles.*

I find some people living in a cabin along the last eight miles of road near the Solomon River amidst winter wilderness. Astonished to see me, they invite me in. The lady seizes my sleeping bag off Hercules and wants to dry it (they have a generator) and says she'll pop it in the dryer. As she makes tea, I go to check it. I open the dryer's door to find feathers everywhere: the sleeping bag is burnt, with a hole two foot wide. I just *can't* let the lady know what's happened. She'd be devastated. I grab a black bag from my kit and stuff the whole lot, feathers and all, into it, cleaning up all the feathers that have escaped everywhere. An old grey dog looks on, wagging his tail as if this were for his enjoyment, sneezing as a feather hits his nose. I pat him, my mind churning. Thinking how I'm to manage now, I drink the tea. I'm so pleased they don't know about it. I thank them for their kindness and leave about half an hour later because I have to fix things up before it gets dark.

I have two other bags but not so warm and tonight I'm cold. The bivvi shakes in the wind and I keep bumping my head, sending ice down onto me as I work to mend the hole in my sleeping bag, which I manage to do with duct tape, Alaska's solution to everything.

The satphone is a lifeline. The batteries have to be nursed, as the solar panel doesn't work in bad weather, but it's set up to do economical emails of up to 60 characters and is invaluable.

I learn that Bob took the tent to be urgently repaired during a quick business trip to Anchorage and is going to try to get it out to me if he can, if the road is open. In an intuitive way he's read my mind, my doubts, observed my living conditions in the bivvi and has taken the initiative. I am so grateful.

Amazingly he makes it through, even though the road has deteriorated, and arrives like Father Christmas, just as

Geoff did in Riga, bringing the tent, perfectly repaired. He's also bought me gloves, five pairs of ice cleats, wonderful dry bags – which are snowproof and waterproof – and many other things. Geoff, Bob and Peter Hutchinson have also apparently been urgently exchanging emails, having been very worried about my burnt sleeping bag, and Peter's making a new one. They are all just great. Bob is the last person I see for 13 days, but I can still see his wry smile at my reaction to his arrival.

Next morning I have to cross a wide, open, frightening-looking stretch of ice leading over the outflow of the Solomon River and inland from shore over the edge of Safety Sound. Patches of water lie everywhere between the ice, some over falls, some very deep. Until you get close up you can't tell which is which, so it's hazardous. It's a mile from the road but could be 100 miles, I feel so remote.

Suddenly there's a deafening roar of wind, from nothing to 75mph. I fall over, cling onto Hercules and stay put. I can't see an inch in front; just hear the crashing of the wind. I burrow my head into my hood and scarves, blessing the mighty Khumbu Gortex and thick down jacket for looking after me as always, and that I'm dressed so warmly with down coat and pants, and waterproof thick storm trousers. I hate being cold and I'm always over the top with warm clothes, but now I appreciate them so much. The big dry bags in the rig are good too as water surges through the ice, splashing up amidst blowing snow. I pray I'm not too near open deep water. I'm shaking with shock and fear, but I found long ago in Russia that fear doesn't matter as long as you keep on doing what you have to do. I have to stay put.

The storm rages; snow piles up against Hercules giving a little shelter. I just curl in a ball and wait, thinking of the story I'd heard, about how the owner of a shack at Solomon went into his shed in a white-out to get firewood and became disorientated. His body was found only 75 yards from his home.

An hour later, just as suddenly as the storm began, it stops. Topkok is infamous for blowholes. The flat area leading from the beach that I'm now on is one of the most dangerous stretches of the Iditarod, but there's no other way to go. It's a good lesson. The ice is cracked in places and I go very, very slowly forward. Now I can see clearly again and I am able to zigzag to avoid the dangers. The new cleats make a big difference in helping me grip the ice. It's hard to pull the load but we've survived the first blowhole intact. I have a vision of brave Hercules who's taken me all through Russia, perched on the gleaming ice of this continent, looking bold in the exquisite evening light that has suddenly spread over the sky. It was his triumphant moment in winter Alaska.

Just before nightfall I get to the main part of the land at last. Exhausted, I put the tent up in the very deep snow. It such a sanctuary – it's like having a fortress compared to the bivouac and I fall asleep in a cocoon of comfort even though it's –30.

CHAPTER 27

Topkok

Alaska, November–December 2005

There's the most blinding, bedazzling beautiful wilderness around Topkok Headland. It's worth everything to see it: the white stretching away with the raging blowing snow of a blowhole just feet ahead, while I'm in total calm. Then I'm hanging on as the space so wide and empty becomes a totally enclosed world, so small I can touch it. The edge of this world is the blowing snow hitting me everywhere, inches from my face. Then it stops and there's majesty and space beyond imagining.

It's worth almost any price and it's not a dream. It's reality. Never was beauty and harshness more closely side by side. I'm soon disappearing up to the waist in the massive drifts of soft powdery snow and Hercules is transformed into an anchor as he sinks deep into the soft snow; the iron frame that's been a source of strength in other situations now drags through the terrain, making it almost impossible for me to move him. Hercules has taken me 10,000 miles, but this terrain is different from any he's encountered in Russia, and he's not built for it. I'm struggling to do 100 yards a day and White Mountain is still 30 miles away. I have to unload

Hercules and carry the bags ahead one at a time. I'm exhausted and very worried.

Day after day I'm struggling to move, pitch the tent, unpitch it, then carry on another 100 yards. I'll never forget the yellow Iditarod trail markers appearing after the white-outs; every one I manage to reach feels like a battle won. It's −25 to −30°C and tiredness makes me feel the cold bitterly, and the tent keeps saving my life. I'm able to get into it with my frozen wet clothes and collapse into the sleeping bags then melt snow-water on the stove and gulp it down as I'm always so thirsty. It's easy to get in a muddle: one day when trying to make a meal I don't put enough snow in the saucepan to cook the spaghetti and it gets stuck to the pan and is almost raw, but I eat it anyway.

I've sent my coordinates on the satphone to Bob who texts me invaluable weather forecasts. I email him that Hercules is having problems with the terrain and that Will Peterson has offered to find me a sled should I need one. I'm hoping for a sled from White Mountain onwards, but Bob knows I'm not moving, saying, 'Not many people understand that northern Alaska *is* Siberia.' The wind screams across the Bering Sea. It's almost December and extremely dangerous. I'm in open wilderness, and hardly moving, so he puts a plan in action to get the sled to me now.

Within a day, in an unbelievable combination of logistics, generosity and caring, Bob calls Will, who contacts well-known walker Denis Douglas, who immediately lends his sled. In a complex flight plan involving two or three differ-ent planes the sled is freighted to Nome. Geoff and Bob guarantee that if the sled is broken or lost by me it will be replaced. Bob puts it on a little plane to White Mountain, hiring two trained White Mountain men, experienced in GPS navigation to stand by at the airport with snowmobiles to transport it to me on the trail.

Hercules has deteriorated. I've been determined some-how to make it with him, but the reality is we're still only doing 100 yards a day. Bob hasn't organised for me to be rescued but has gone to far greater efforts to help me continue. He's saved the whole project. I *have* to get to White Mountain on foot: the promise I made in running around the world for cancer awareness after Clive died is that I would do it all on foot – or even crawl on all fours as I have occasionally had to do up steep hills or risk falling backwards into the ravines.

The times that I am loneliest for my family and friends are when I am having a few days' rest. Like all experienced adventurers – when I was sailing around Cape Horn or going solo across the Atlantic and now – the total focus is on how to cope and survive. Fear is a luxury: when you are in a really dangerous situation you cannot let yourself become too frightened because otherwise you can't think clearly and you have to think clearly to be able to cope and get yourself out of all challenging situations. These are my personal beliefs but they are also common-sense general rules for everybody facing any major problems.

It's mid-morning on 30 November. I hear them a long time before I see them. There's a high-pitched whining and screaming of snowmobiles, their riders silhouetted on top of a drift against the skyline, and then zooming down towards me. Moments later, Dean Pushruk and Chris Nassuk from White Mountain are alongside me, beaming and saying, 'Hello, lady, how are you?'

It's exciting to see them. They say it's taken eight hours to get here over terrain they describe as very rough and nasty. One of them has damaged the track on his snowmobile, lost his face-mask and goggles. It's extremely hard-going. Dean says that the same trip, if taken later in the winter on a broken packed trail, would normally take about 45 minutes.

They lift the sled off their trailer. It's pretty-looking with a yellow canopy over it in which I can rest, sleep and live. As well as the sled, Dean and Chris have brought fuel for my tiny stove, extra food and a handheld CB radio, the standard form of communication between villages and people on the trail. Fred Ross, a teacher at White Mountain School, lends me his snowshoes. They say the whole village of 250 people are aware of my trek and everyone is longing to meet me.

They leave, taking Hercules and 90lb of equipment back to White Mountain. Because the new system is more simple I don't have the big tent now, nor the mats, groundsheets, tarps and so on. I have just the little dry bags, as my big heavy ones won't fit in this sled, and I don't need them. Nothing is taken out of the tent, since it's situated on the sled and just stays there as always. Aerodynamically it's so good, as I soon discover: the wind just shafts over it like an aeroplane wing. Throughout the whole of my run, one thing I've learnt is that the weather can be utterly ruthless. The bivvi has saved my life, as did the Quasar tent recently, especially during the last few days. But now I can leave the sleeping bags unrolled on the bed in the sled and just get in without having to fight to put up a shelter with frozen hands or when I'm exhausted. Though it is small, only 6ft by 30in, I can lie in it full length.

The route around the ravine is steep, with inclines down and up through gulleys and frozen creeks, and difficult areas with willow brush among the snowdrifts. The sled follows fairly willingly and I can even lift it over some of the worst obstacles. I manage about four miles a day – which is *flying* compared to my previous progress.

After five days I'm approaching White Mountain village along a frozen river. It looks bleak. I can just make out small buildings high up on the bank. Then I see a little girl in a bright red snowsuit, alone on the river ice. I wonder what she's doing out there all by herself. She looks at me and smiles then raises her hand and waves.

Suddenly a crowd of children, laughing and cheering, come rushing from where they've been hiding to surprise me. They're holding an enormous banner saying:

'WHITE MOUNTAIN ALASKA – WELCOME ROSIE!'

CHAPTER 28

White Mountain

Alaska, December 2005

The children want me to run through the banner like the tape at the end of a marathon, but it's much too beautiful for that and I'll always treasure it.

White Mountain is magical, like its name. I stay there three happy days. Andy Haviland, the School Principal, and the villagers can't do more for me. I'm able to check all my equipment and pick up my snowshoes and ice shovel that have been sent here; and Bee Gee, a lady reindeer herder, gives me a reindeer skin for the sled. The school also agrees to keep Hercules in their heated workshop to be sent on later when I reach the road system.

Before I leave, Joanna Wassillie, one of the teachers, says: 'Rosie, when you see a star, remember they're the same stars we look at and that we're thinking of you. That way you'll know you're never alone.' The school's ski team escort me down the river before saying farewell.

There's something so special about the Eskimo villages along the Bering Sea coast stretching ahead over the next 200 miles – Golovin, Elim, Shaktooklik, Unalakleet. It's to do with their powerful sense of caring community. Their environment is unspeakably cruel and remote. In a situation where people can die just yards from home in the cold, a mile is a long way and the 40–60 miles between villages can seem like 1000 miles. They depend on each other because they have to. They have more materially than the Russians but that doesn't alter the weather which is even harsher. Here the terrain is impassable nine or ten months of the year. The villages are islands in the midst of ice and storms and whiteness in winter, and amid swamps and tundra in summer. The only way out usually is by air, if weather permits. They couldn't survive without this closeness of community, and a stranger like me who arrives even briefly is embraced into it, and the memory of it sees you through the wilderness beyond.

I run a few miles along the firm ice of Golovin Bay and then climb up into the mountains on a winter trail over a big headland to get to Norton Sound.

Four days later, it's gusting 60–70mph. The wind is like a wall hitting you. I skid backwards, I'm thrown into a pile of snowdrifts and brushwood, and stay there for four days. I crawl into the sled. I can't go forwards or backwards. I dig the sled out at intervals, or I'd not only have been buried but packed in tight in the drift, as the snow is wild and thick and comes in and beats down with violence. I just lie there, that's all I can do. I later hear that this storm has affected the whole state. I learn to use the stove very carefully inside the tiny sled: I need to melt snow to drink and eat as it's now impossible outside. I'm absolutely focused on the little flame. My diet is tea, and spaghetti mixed with reindeer hairs, as my reindeer skin begins shedding and I can never get them all out, but it doesn't seem to do my insides any harm so far as I can tell. It will be another recipe for that cookbook.

When the storm ends about 19 December, I set off along the last few miles to Norton Sound over a landscape of huge new drifts transformed by the crazy artistry of the wind. I descend to the shore a day afterwards and gaze at the endless-looking ice of the big bay. I feel almost like an ancient explorer, that maybe I've crossed not only from Golovin Bay but perhaps over a continent and epoch to reach this shore, and that I'm the first ever to look out over it. I think I've lost my brain in the storm. I've only come 40 miles from White Mountain in the last eleven days. Wales and the Bering Strait are still only 290 miles back and it's taken over two months to get from there.

There's a good route along the sea-ice to Elim, and the last message from Elim on the two-way radio says the ice is still solid after the storm. Suddenly I have a very bad feeling about it. I've heard nothing more. There's no signal on the radio and the satphone is flat (the batteries have been wiped by the cold). The sky is now brighter, so I get out the solar panel and sit by the shore, recharging the phone; after an hour there's one bar on the battery and I see an urgent message. Bob has emailed: the local people have repeatedly tried to call me on the two-way radio to warn me the sea-ice has 'blown out' and separated from the shore-ice. If I go further, I'll be adrift on an iceberg or floe, broken off from the main body of the ice with no way back.

There are no atheists on an adventure or in battle. I reckon it's time to say thank you to God, to all those caring for me, and the *Runner's World* satphone that has saved me and is to save me again.

CHAPTER 29

Breaking the Ice

Alaska, December 2005–January 2006

I find a way through inland behind Haystack Mountain. Like a breath amid the struggles, I spend Christmas and a few days of calm at the village of Elim, cherishing the memories: people bringing their presents to church to be opened together, a Native Alaskan custom; children's big eyes; being able to call my four-year-old grandson Michael from a landline through Elim's tiny telephone exchange; how Andrea and May, two teenage girls, bring a small tree specially for my cabin; a two-week-old husky puppy setting off by himself in the snow and being taken back home; and breakfast on my last day with a villager called Oscar, his wife and ten children. 'The Good Lord did tell us "Go forth be fruitful and multiply",' says Oscar.

It's my third Christmas away. I do not think any longer after all this time about lost Christmases – I think of the future. And the fact that all the people I meet who share so much with me will also be part of the life of my family and me in all the years that may lie ahead of us.

It's a fairly straightforward 48 miles along a smooth stretch of shore-ice to Koyuk, where New Year becomes another happy memory. Wayne comes out on his snowmobile as I approach the village, bringing his wife Fanny's hot soup and stew, and packing the trail for me, so I can run in more easily. Inviting me to attend the New Year's Day service I fall asleep for an hour and a half behind a pew. Fannie makes me a bed on the floor with a jacket, because the sermon is three hours long. I have to confess to the Pastor afterwards, but he's very forgiving.

On 2 January I set off on the 55 miles mostly on the sea-ice to Shaktoolik en route to Unalakleet, the only way to get there. I'm walking at night when the wind drops, but although there's no wind, the ice is shaking under my feet, reverberating to what sounds like explosions or thunderbolts, which is the ice crashing together somewhere out in the bay. It's a primitive, terrifying noise, deafening, even from afar. I can see nothing on this dark night as I shine the torch, taking one step at a time as there's a white-out suspended like a wall beneath the darkness. But it's the noise that fills my head. The weather forecast says the wind will blow the ice north, not towards me. I *am* making progress. There's no safety for anybody who travels on this ice: it can get you at any time, but I'm as safe as it's possible to be in this situation. I owe everything to the people of Koyuk who've given me a careful course along the ice, not too far out in the bay.

'The wind from Siberia shifts and pushes the sea-ice up against the shore-ice,' I'm told. 'It just piles up against itself and can be hundreds of feet high. The sea-ice crushes the shore-ice and the various plates of ice are moving across the surface, crashing into each other. If you're out in this, it's hard to say which would be worse: breaking off on the ice and floating out to sea, with the hope you'll float back, or being caught out when it's piling on top of you.'

At daybreak, the wind starts blasting in. It's uneconomical in terms of my own energy to keep struggling and I have to get some sleep so I can go on again the next night. It's shift-work. I have to figure out how to stop the sled disappearing out to sea with me in it while I'm asleep. It's so lightweight and there's nothing to tie it to, no shelter. I'm out on the exposed open sea.

The extraordinary thing is the aerodynamic miracle that made this little sled so good to start with can be made here to work to keep it still. It can be sort of 'hove to' like a little boat on a voyage. I use much the same method and put the sled nose to the wind and for good measure lay the equipment bags roped together all around the sled so the snow may be caught and trapped and build up in a drift around us. This way, the tiny sled just sits there even in a 50mph wind. I just can't believe it. It makes all the difference because otherwise I wouldn't get sleep or rest or do my cooking or navigation.

I always take my coordinates on the GPS before 'bedtime' and recheck my position when I awake, desperately hoping I haven't drifted all the way back to Siberia.

Later I'm asked, '*How* did you spend all those hours alone in the sled. Did you read a good book? Did you listen to music? The hours must have seemed like eternity.'

But it isn't like that at all. It's a struggle to do all the things I have to do. As well as the specific challenges of being on the ice on the sea, it's still −35, and so looking after my hands, as usual, makes everything slow. I'm doing things in slow motion again because I'm clumsy in the cold, and it's quite hard, with wind buffeting the canvas, to do chores and errands: set up the solar panel in bright calm moments; pick up the weather forecasts on the satphone from Bob who's sending them through thick and thin; plot them into the log; try to get reports on the two-way radio; keep clean and occasionally mend the kit, and so on. The rest of the time I sleep because it's very tiring. So even roaring wind by day, and crashing ice day and night while I'm on the bay, can't stop me sleeping sounder than a baby.

One of the radio reports speaks of rescue helicopters having been called out by some people adrift on the ice further in the bay. When the Rescue Services got there, the ice has drifted back in, and they're OK, but it must have been a very harrowing experience.

At last on 6 January I make it across the bay, pulling my sled onto the frozen tundra on solid land. I feel like leaping for joy.

CHAPTER 30

Crazy Rogue

Alaska, January–February 2006

'Great to see you again, you Crazy Rogue!' shouts Ferno affectionately after she rushes out to meet me as I reach Unalakleet. 'Finally, someone even crazier than me.'

It feels like a lifetime since I was here on the way to Wales with Ferno's brother, Dr Adrian Ryan. On my run I'm always saying goodbye so it's great seeing Eva and Ferno and their family again. I think I'll do the run again just to revisit everyone. It's also goodbye to the Bering Sea, after over 300 miles of the coastline. On 13 January I set off inland along the old Kaltag Portage Trail that leads for 90 miles through the mountains to link the Bering Sea with the Yukon River. I've been warned it's going to be much colder inland.

Two days after I leave Unalakleet an exceptional spell of –60 and –65°C begins, lasting nine days.

15 January: The cold is uncanny. Nothing moves. There's no sound. For days I haven't seen a bird or animal. Nothing is around when it's this cold. There's no snowmobile traffic from the villages as the engines would freeze. Not a breath of wind either. Even the wind has submitted as if frozen or

overawed. The silence is surreal. Icy whiteness has taken over the whole world.

Survival takes up all my time. This is another occasion when the situation is too serious to allow fear to take over. I have to think clearly. I'll never forget the first time I wake in the sled, my heart thundering, I don't know why. I realise I'm shaking too. It's *very cold*. I shine the torch and the thermometer inside is reading –62. I *mustn't* sleep until I get warmer.

By day, progress is so slow. The snow is deep, and around 1pm the temperature drops dramatically. It's so tempting to go on but the difference between managing in normal cold and this is that even an extra five minutes out in the snow can be the difference between life and death.

When it gets that cold you can't control your hands and then you can't *do* anything. In this temperature your hands are equally as important as your feet. Without the use of them, you're completely helpless.

So this becomes the routine: I haul the sled to the side of the trail in the deep snow; make a grab for the zip of the tent entrance and somehow force it open, undo the straps of my snowshoes and plunge inside, shutting the flap. Everything in the sled is frozen solid and soon starts to melt with my body warmth. I fight to get the boots off, rubbing my feet as hard as I can, then get into the sleeping bags. They're wet, sodden and icy. The salvation is the two beautiful tanned reindeer skins my friend Bob sent to Unalakleet for me. They're the secret of survival among Native Alaskans for hundreds of years. They're damp but I hang them out for an instant in the cold. The hair freezes and I can then knock off the droplets by hand and the skin is dry again. I wrap one around me in the sleeping bags and put the other one under me.

The first urgent job is to get something hot to eat and drink. The only difference from usual is that I have to light a small candle before nursing the stove to life – a highly dangerous manoeuvre with all my possessions already occupying most of the 6ft by 30in space, but necessary as the matches are damp. Anyway, I have wonderful coffee and spaghetti.

I still feel very cold but eventually the sleeping bags puff out and I'm warm enough to be able to put my damp socks and insoles in the bag to dry out for the morning. Then I sleep to be ready for the next day.

It's a beautiful trail, still utterly deserted. I'm frightened yet privileged to be here alone. The lovely trees are now covered in ice like a shroud but the day before I get to Kaltag, one bird – about thrush size, of the kind they call 'camp robbers' – hops down from a tree in front of me. It's the first living creature I've seen for six days. It means the worst of the cold is over for now.

It's a great moment when I finally arrive on the western shore of Yukon River which is much wider than I expected. It begins snowing and I can't see the shores either side, but ahead of me on the river are large uninhabited islands appearing out of the mists and snow, as if they rather than I had just arrived there. The snow above the ice is deep, but there are some old snowmobile tracks and they're like gold dust, because I can pull the sled more easily. The temperature has risen to about –30. The trail is harder and better frozen at night. So once again everything has changed and I carry on a lot again after dark. It's back on the night-shift.

On 2 February I arrive at the Athabascan Native Alaskan village of Nulato. It's snowing heavily and just before night-fall I'm pulling the sled along the little street, unsure where to go, when a man outside the church comes up to greet me. It turns out to be the Franciscan Friar, Brother Bob. Within minutes he's taken charge of the sled and has pulled it right into the little church. Two other very elderly men, waiting for the service, retrieve all my smelly, wet, soggy equipment, sleeping bags and reindeer skins from the sled and spread them all over the pews to dry.

The sled stays in the church all the time I'm in the village. It's a truly Christian thing to do. Brother Bob is loved by everyone in the village, even those who don't attend church. He also does haircuts. He's very proud of the 'barber's kit' his brother sent him from Connecticut. People are queuing next day to have their hair done and I think, *Oh I'll have a trim too.* He's not shy with the scissors. He takes one look at my scraggly locks and they're gone. I look in my little mirror in my wash bag and decide I won't get any calls from *Vogue*.

Steven Seaton has flown out from Britain to check I'm OK and take photos. The last time I saw him was a year and a half ago in Omsk. It's fabulous to see him. My route is developing and the decision is made to run along the River Yukon to Tanana then head for Fairbanks, instead of going south and up again from Anchorage as it's a more direct way.

The Athabascan Indian old-timers I meet in Nulato inform me that the heart won't rest when it's as cold as this. I understand now about the pounding of my heart that first time I awoke in the sled in the bitter cold: it was nature's way of keeping me awake in case I never wake up. They teach me how to shove handfuls of dried grass, stored from summer, down my front for insulation, advising me to drink gallons of fish oil to keep warm, and just get on with life. They're tough people – Nulato, far from any roads, has a reputation for wildness and shootings – but very hospitable. Loyalty is the keynote of their lives.

It's such fun to give a talk at Nulato School. I'm staying with a teacher, Joyce Metza. The pupils are tough kids from hard homes and Joyce thinks the world of them. The Principal agrees I should do the talk but not expect any questions. However, it turns out Joyce has primed her class with all the stories about the 'Man with the Axe' and so on in Russia. To my great surprise after talking I'm inundated with very interesting questions from all sides of the room.

'Tell us about the Naked Man with the Gun,' says one big boy.

'Did the wild dogs bite your bottom, miss?' says another, aged about eight.

The Principal is stunned and the boy is removed from the room. But Joyce Metza is smiling. She tells me this little boy rarely speaks – and has *never* asked a question before. I get a message later that the boy seldom stops talking now since his bold question has made him famous amongst his mates. He's doing better at his school-work too. If only the wild dogs of Russia could have known what effect they've had on this child.

CHAPTER 31

The Comeback

Alaska, February–April 2006

It's been blowing snow all night. The sled is half-buried – and me with it – but it's no problem to dig it out with my faithful ice shovel. The snow lifts and swirls above the river in a dance with snowflakes that start falling from the sky once more, but it's only –15.

Extreme cold of –60°C alternating with –15 or –20 means exceptionally dangerous conditions everywhere. Richard Strick, one of the community of Ruby, a village I passed through a week ago, has been killed by an avalanche, caused by unstable snow while packing a trail in the mountains for the forthcoming Iron Dog Race, which is an epic snowmobile race that takes place in Alaska. It was heartbreaking and I'm dedicating this part of the run to him.

I've become preoccupied with following little snowy ridges, the only remaining signs of a track. Markers are few, and deceptive when they've been there all winter. Far beneath its burdens of deep, soft snow and jammed, sharp icebergs, the ice is alive. It can move around with a will of its own. Today's safe route can become tomorrow's disaster. Finding a snowmobile track, even faint, is priceless – and greatly adds to all the information I receive from the GPS. The Yukon is a mile wide here, but in bad visibility might as well be as big as an ocean; and the wild uninhabited islands, sloughs and tributaries are dim ghosts that come and go.

Eventually I stop, having made it from Hardluck Island – whose name should have been a warning – to Florence Island. Immediately, I realise something is very wrong. When I try to haul off my boots after tumbling into the sled, I can't. The ice around my left foot is set so solidly I have to use my knife to hack off the sock. Water has penetrated the boots and refrozen on my feet.

The right foot is OK, but the big toe on the left foot is deep purple with a blister on it twice the size of the toe. I'm outraged with myself. My ethics, my absolute conviction, my *law*, almost my religion from the very start of the journey when I left Tenby and realised I wasn't coming back and had nowhere to recover, has been to avoid injury. I've been nearly fanatical about it and haven't even had any normal blisters, until now – and nothing can change it back to how it was before.

Then I think, *Maybe it's not too bad*. I call Bob and explain I have minor frostbite. He's very worried but I say I'm OK. He reads the first-aid instructions for frostbite treatment down the crackly satphone connection from his medical manual. Most of all, it's about what *not* to do:

Do not rub
Above all, do not thaw slowly.
Frostbite has to be thawed fast …

It recommends putting the toe or damaged area into warm water, 104–108°F (40–42°C).

I melt the snow, forgetting all about the coffee, and heat the water and stick my toe in the saucepan. I email that I'm absolutely fine. The toe is agony now it's thawed, which I take as a good sign. I swallow Ibuprofen which I hardly ever take. It sends me soundly to sleep, pain or no. By morning, the foot is still warm, hasn't refrozen, though the blister is large and disgusting-looking, as if a giant deep-purple slug or leech had stuck onto my toe.

'Frostbite in big toe still there, but not worse,' I email. 'Feet wrapped in fur and drybags within Native Mukluk boots. Determined to get to Tanana.'

I *have* to get going. It's 80–100 miles to the village, but I think I can make it, slowly, just a few miles a day. I wrap the foot in beaver fur underneath my socks and boots to prevent the blister bursting, and set off.

Snow is blowing again. There's no visibility, no trail, just deep snow, but I can keep going. I carry on like this for two days. 'Take five steps. *Stop!* Take ten steps. *Stop!* Think of my family. Sing "All Things Bright and Beautiful".' If I'm not going to need treatment for frostbite, I'm definitely going to need it for my head.

It's a great break on 24 February to see a snowmobile, one of a team packing the trail in preparation for the Serum Run. This is an annual dog-team journey with snowmobile support across 786 miles from Nenana to Nome that celebrates the courageous mushers and dogs who were part of the Great Race of Mercy in 1925, when dog teams took the vital diphtheria serum to Nome during the epidemic, saving the population.

It's a rare sunny clear day, with lightly blowing snow over the river. Spectacular to see beautiful huskies racing towards me. Kurt, the musher, stops his dogs, smiles, says hello and starts chatting.

'You'd better not stop to talk to me,' I say, 'you're in the *lead*.'

'This isn't a race,' he replies. 'It's something more than that.' He says that many of the mushers on the original run succumbed to frostbite, and some of the dogs had died, but the serum got there through their heroism.'

I explain what I'm doing. Then all the teams come into view and stop, handing me biscuits and chocolates from the bib pockets around their necks. The huskies have polar fleece bootees on their paws to protect them and are keen to get going. Two weeks ago in Ruby I met Emmitt Peters, 'The Yukon Fox', who won the Iditarod as a rookie, because his dogs, led by his leader Nugget, kept running even after he'd fallen asleep from exhaustion in a storm halfway across Norton Sound. Just to see the enthusiasm and spirit of the huskies here does the heart good.

One musher is a nurse who wants to check my frostbite but it's impossible in the blowing snow in the open. 'Take great care,' she says, asking if I have antibiotics. I reply I carry Amoxillin as I have trouble with my teeth, and she tells me this isn't good for frostbite, and if it starts to smell, call for help. I hope to have the frostbite treated at the next village. Tanana is now only 55 miles away. The trail the sleds and snowmobiles have packed down is a great boost, a total gift for my foot. I should make it now without trouble to Tanana.

I go to bed happy and elated, sleeping very well because of the painkillers. I don't hear the storm starting. By morning it's blizzard conditions: five foot of new snow have fallen during the night and it's –55°C. There's no sign left of a trail or that the dog run ever passed by. I walk on for another day, thinking every mile makes a difference, but soon have to stop for a long time as the storm is so severe. I suppose the rest in the sled will help the foot anyway.

But the next day, the toe gets much worse. By the following day I can't walk, because it's swollen too much to get my boot on. I have no clean dressings left; everything is becoming chaotic: the bandages have reindeer hair stuck to them. I don't dare step outside and put weight on the foot, as a rash – a sign of possible gangrene – and the blister is oozing and beginning to burst.

I call Bob with my coordinates but he's much more worried about the toe. He can't call me on my sat system but asks me to phone back. The doctors he's consulted are extremely concerned that I'm in danger of losing a toe, foot or leg or worse. I want to wait the toe out, but the reality is I can't.

We discuss getting help or medicine to me from Tanana, but the storm will make it extremely hazardous for villagers' snowmobiles now. It's just blowing up and up. I now understand why people put things off, why they try to overlook things and keep going. I hate needing help so much. If I died in Russia in the wilds, that would have been unfortunate; I had eaten berries and tree bark to survive. Now that I have a way of surviving and finishing the journey, by getting the necessary medical treatment, I must do it. It's as stark as that.

And the thing that will stop everything is pride – or the false pride that's my weakness; I *have* to beat myself. Just as I've walked on with frostbite while I could, I have to take the help now that I can get it. I've never asked for help even when sailing the Atlantic solo years ago and the boat nearly capsized, but if I don't take the right decision now, I'll be culpable in my mind. The run's loss will be my fault. I'll brand myself a coward in my mind for ever if I'm stupid and don't have the strength to face my physical vulnerability – and the pain of not always getting my own way.

I owe everything to Bob and the Alaska National Guard for the events that follow. To start with, it's the deep respect I have for Bob for making me listen. Bittersweet as it is, if I want to continue my journey, my foot has to be saved.

I put my strobe-light out and give Bob and the Alaska National Air Guard team my exact coordinates. I'm camped beside yet another uninhabited impenetrable island called Henry Island at N64 00. 946 W154 02.455. They're there within 90 minutes. I speak to those coming to get me on the satphone, hear their voices on the phone and then the roaring of helicopters above me. The Arctic storm is raging all the while. Four bright red flares are dropped near my strobe-light. The helicopter briefly lands; the men come running over to get me. I'm soon looking into the kind, smiling faces of John Romspert and his team.

They take me and the sled to Anchorage, involving the aerial refuelling of the helicopter in gale-force winds before landing in Galana, and switching to a Hercules aircraft because the weather is so severe they can't take me to Fairbanks, which is much closer. They're amazing. I have more medical attention in the helicopter in the blizzard than ever before in my life. They care for me non-stop, packing my foot with warm bags, putting a saline drip in my arm, offering morphine, constantly checking my blood pressure, and much more. They're caring, brave and gallant. I'll never forget the pilot or the team, John, Steven, Romero and Mario.

'Even a racing car needs a pit-stop,' Major Mike Haller greets me when we reach Anchorage. The modern equipment two-way radio, satphone and GPS have made their job 'easy' in the horrific weather. My insurance agent, Joshua Weinstein in Anchorage, phones to say I'm fully covered, but for all the extraordinary efforts they've made the Alaska National Air Guard won't take any money. They say it's a 'training exercise'. *Some training exercise.* If my mishap and the publicity give me a chance to thank them better and reinforce the fact that these wonderful people risk their lives for others every day and that they must be appreciated, not only when they are needed, but always, then my frostbite will have been worthwhile.

The Providence Hospital frostbite specialist says I can't continue for at least six months: I could lose the big toe or it will never be the same again. 'They make very good shoes,' he adds. 'Nobody will know.' It's very depressing.

I'm determined after all the help I've received to return to the coordinates where I was picked up and resume my run from there, to keep faith with the world track and my promises, especially as I've added the Alaska National Air

Guard's personal charity to my special causes. They dress up as elves and fly to remote Eskimo and Athabascan village to deliver gifts for the children before Christmas. I've been there and met those villagers. For this reason alone I'm intent on making it back on the ice. The big problem is I must get back to the Yukon before the ice breaks up in five weeks, or wait a year as the terrain on the banks is impassable. To wait a year will end the journey in the spirit in which it's being done, which though slow has been non-stop.

It seems impossible but I do make it back in four weeks – thanks to the exceptional, compassionate, expert care I receive from so many people, including Dr Carolyn Craig and the advice from the National Guard Medics, who don't see obstacles in the same way as anyone else. My toe is saved.

On 2 April, with my foot still wrapped in bandages as a precaution, I board a commercial flight to Fairbanks with the sled, and take another small aeroplane to Tanana. The ice is still intact and the weather has improved. The Tanana villagers, who are there for me body and soul, arrange for someone to haul the sled and me by snowmobile those 55 vital miles back to Henry Island.

At 2pm on 4 April I reach Henry Island. We cross my track plus an extra mile for luck. The kind villager signs a piece of paper verifying the time, date and place, and gives me a delicious bag of smoked salmon bits for treats. Soon he's just a speck and then he's gone.

*   *   *

The distance from here to Tanana, which seemed as far as the moon when I had the frostbite, is now fairly straightforward. I manage about ten miles a day, which surprises me as my foot still has a light bandage on it. But the sled is not as heavy as usual because I don't need so many stores for this short distance.

I run at night under the light of the Aurora Borealis. The whole ice-cape of the river and the banks beyond reflects the exquisite colours of orange, green, scarlet and aquamarine, as the Aurora swirls and dances across the night sky. The wolves howl from the banks of the Yukon, as if the Aurora had disturbed them or awoken ancient feelings. I think of the wolves of Siberia, and how lucky I am to have known all this on my run. I've been given a second chance after the frostbite. I'll make the most of it and keep on doing the very best I can. I never will get over why people are always so good to me.

On the fifth day, I see dots hurtling towards me from far away on the ice. It's all the villagers coming out on their snowmobiles to meet me. They take my sled for the last few miles. I've removed the bandages off my foot by now so for the first time in months I *run free*. I nearly sprint through the snow those final miles to Tanana. It's incredible that I've made it before the ice breaks up.

Tanana is a village with a school, two churches and a small shop owned by Cynthia and Dale. What's special and poignant is that this is the last village on my run to which no road leads because of the terrain and conditions. There's something unique not in circumstance alone, but in spirit, about those villages to which no roads go, from Wales to Tanana. They'll always be in my heart.

A last stretch across the Yukon, down the Tanana River and along Fish Creek, a wilderness full of hoof- and paw-prints in the snow and signs of bears waking up. Just before I get to the end of this, on the final part of wilderness, I fall on blue ice and break a few ribs. In comparison with frost-bite, it's nothing. The hardship of the journey is changing my perspective on obstacles, making them seem less, but above all I'm reminded that the real battle of life is that fought and endured by people with cancer and similar illnesses and others like the orphans of Kitezh. I tell *everybody* about my mission wherever I go and I hope it helps. I'm powerfully aware, now as always, that my run is *for* Clive but not *about* Clive. He has given me my life back and this is the best way to pay him respect, honour and love.

Suddenly on 12 April, near a tiny goldmine marked on the map as Tofty, I'm in another world. I reach a *road*.

CHAPTER 32

Reunion

Alaska–Canada, May–June 2006

Instead of ice, snow, and desolation, blinding white-outs and temperatures of –60, it's the fever of the short blazing summer of Alaska. I'm on the Alaska Highway near the Canadian border in June, awaiting the greatest moment of my journey. I'm going to see my son. I'll be able to hold James, talk to him. I'll never ever take anything like this for granted after this run. I haven't seen him since the day I left Tenby, two and a half years ago, the day of the first step engraved into my flagstone, of the uneaten birthday cake when I was suddenly gone around the first corner, cheered by family and friends as if it were just a little run and they were expecting me back for breakfast. It seems like a lifetime ago and like no time at all. The excitement is unbearable ...

Runner's World have sponsored James's visit. It's just one of their extraordinary gifts. I hardly know what to do with myself on 12 June. It's a beautiful, crazy day even before he gets here. Early morning I wash my hair in a lake – I want to look my best. Now I can wash in lakes and rivers, I try to be economical with shampoo, to avoid disturbing the tadpoles and other lake residents. This time it definitely works, because while my head is stuck in water I see schools of minnows, beetles and whirring insects darting around near my ears. I hope they won't nip and swish them away.

A little later I'm running down the road and a *fish* jumps out of my hair. I wonder if I've finally lost my mind. But the fish *is* there, wriggling on the road. I pick him up. 'Don't worry, you're too small to eat.'

I put him in the water-bottle; he's swimming frantically. You can't go fly-fishing with your hair as the line. I take him back to his lake – a matter of honour and a distraction for my pent-up excitement – and watch him swim away free. He's the little one that got away.

The big moment draws close around midday. I'm near a town called Tok, my stomach churning; every minute is an hour. I have balloons tied to the cart and a large 'ROSIE IS HERE!' sign. I *can't* let them miss me. Suddenly a car comes into view, stops and James gets out, looking the same as ever, tall and handsome. He's slightly built with gentle manners and ways, but indefatigable, steely determination combined with a dry sense of humour. James and Eve have been with me throughout the journey in spirit in a way that has made all the difference. I can't believe he's here.

With James in the car is Abigail Neal, a young BBC Wales reporter who's fought hard to get a commission to come out with James. Apparently lots of people in Wales have been concerned about the frostbite. The people of Tok have arranged a fabulous welcome and a concert of traditional songs by great local singers. We stay at Don and Barb Abbott's campsite, the Tundra RV Park, and Abigail comes camping too. We have a happy evening under the trees, cooking supper on the camping stove and catching up on stories. Just seeing photos of Michael and family and friends, and hearing stories about Tenby from Abigail, makes me realise my painful hunger for news. Knowing James is in the tent next to me I am too excited to sleep. My mind goes back over the past six weeks ...

The sled had come to a full stop when I'd arrived at the road. It had been such a friend, I wouldn't risk it for a mile along the gritty verge of the ploughed road that could damage it in a way that even the 70mph storms in Norton Bay hadn't done. It was indeed a little sled with a giant heart. At Tofty, I'd met Bunny, a solitary goldminer, driving an earth-moving machine up an impossible-looking mud mountain. He'd taken the sled and my kit to his house in Manley 20 miles along my route. From there it was returned to Denis Douglas with my grateful thanks.

Bunny's girlfriend Carole, a health-aid worker in Manley, examined the dark-blue swollen bruise on my side where the ribs had broken. You could see the ends of the ribs wobbling. I was bored by being injured. Getting to the road had been my big goal. 'Yesterday's hardship is today's anaes-thetic.' I stayed with them for several days with an ice-pack on the ribs. Bunny fixed up an old pushchair attaching an iron bar as a shaft so I could pull it from Manley to Fair-banks. Carole gave me a sheepskin to put round the bar so it didn't hurt too much, another bag of painkillers and I set off slowly for the city, arriving 5 May. At Fairbanks, I received generous hospitality from Brother Bob's friends, the Reverend Sisters of Fairbanks Diocese, who looked after me while my ribs healed. I remember the kindness of Sister Dorothy, known as Princess Polar Bear, who loves the bush and wolves, and there were many others.

I was privileged to meet Karl Bushby and Dimitri Kieffer shortly after their epic crossing of the Bering Strait. I'd nearly met Karl on Norton Bay, where we had missed each other because of bad weather, passing like ships in the night. But they'd driven out on the road to meet me near Fairbanks, bringing good wishes through Karl's father Keith. They've inspired me even more to cross the Bering Strait on the ice myself – my next dream.

The saddest news in Fairbanks was that the beautiful White Mountain School had burnt in an accidental fire two months before. The brave ski team whom I'd met had won the school championships with borrowed kit, all their equipment having been destroyed. Hercules had been presumed burnt, though thankfully no lives had been lost. But the story wasn't over. The school had been magnificently rebuilt – and Hercules had been found. Bob Collins was determined to get him back for me and so Hercules (now known as Lazarus!) had been sent by DHL to Fairbanks to replace the old pushchair. I'd pulled him 180 miles from Fairbanks to Tok and my rendezvous with James.

*   *   *

Hercules is as fine as ever. He could have continued around the world now I'm back on the road, but the sled's inbuilt tent has been such an advantage. So *Runner's World* has commissioned Steve Holland and Giles Dyson to make me a new buggy, canopy and all. It was delivered to Tok the day before James and I arrived. We are going to open it on our first day together. Bearing in mind Hercules is so strongly built – he survived a bus crash as well as the fire – it's no surprise the Silver Dream Machine, by the same designer, is substantial. It weighs in with my possessions at 252lb on the local weighbridge, but is immaculately designed. It looks spectacular, silver and sparkling in the sunshine, made of composites with a big bar around it and three wheels and a cute green tent on top. It takes practice to get used to it, but the three-wheel system is marvellous as it takes the weight off my shoulders. The campsite owners have offered to take Hercules safely to Anchorage to Bob's cabin at Wasilla for a well-earned retirement.

I continue to the Canadian border with James and Abigail, and when she has to return to Wales, James takes over their hire car and we have another wonderful fortnight together. While I run through the day, James is sightseeing, making trips to Fairbanks to get equipment and bits and pieces. He returns every night to cook. It's such fun to wake up and say, 'Good morning, how did you sleep?' to another human being, especially my own son. To discuss the day, talk about the beautiful scenery as we carry on into Canada, sharing little everyday things, means so much to me. We meet fascinating people at the campsites, including a man who's had a heart attack and didn't know about it for six months, leaving him with a damaged heart. He could die any time but was still achieving his dream of cycling across Canada and Alaska.

James is a great chef. As I'm running on the road every day, I look forward so much to seeing him waiting along the verge around midday with the camping stove out, steam rising from the saucepan as he cooks yet another delicious meal. I've become fitter and stronger during these two weeks than ever before. I'm sure I've put on half a stone.

James's visit gave me so much mental strength and after his return to the UK, I carry on through the summer knowing he's with me in every way, and maintaining the website as always. Through his visit, the pictures, my grandson's video and our conversations, the whole family, all of us, are now even closer.

CHAPTER 33

Ballad of the
Red Toenails

Canada—United States, July 2006—June 2007

The next few months are a swathe of easy running along the
Alcan Highway through Canada in lovely summer weather,
on average about 16 miles a day. I pass Liard Hot Springs,
with warm bubbling mineral water and friendly travellers
and notices like The Mosquitoes Prayer: 'Please send more
tourists, the last ones were delicious'; and see shaggy herds of
buffalo and grizzly bears unperturbed in the forest near the
roadside, often peaceably grazing on berries, occasionally
standing up and towering unbelievably tall. They lazily
yawn, revealing teeth that seem inches long, as are their
claws. Being used to people doesn't make them less dangerous, but they're magnificent and mostly attack when startled. That's why hikers wear bearbells, but I've got my little
cassette recorder and am entertaining the grizzlies to Strauss
and Billy Joel.

I follow my wilderness rules: Saying I *can* takes no more
breath than saying I *can't*. Never stop halfway up a hill –
only when you're over the top. Leave space and energy to
deal with anything unexpected that happens. When times
are difficult, think of something very special to keep you

going: you can be the most decadent person in your mind eating chocolates, or out with someone you love when you're struggling and fighting to survive at –50°C.

It's steep and mountainous on the edge of the Rockies. Occasionally I have to cling to trees to prevent myself rolling back with the rig, but the run's relatively simple compared with the past. Yet sometimes it's 'hard when it's easy' with a lot of time to reflect. I keep thinking, *Help! I've been running around the world for three years non-stop!* There's still so far to go. I believe that if you can keep your strength in a difficult situation, that strength is still yours for ever when you need it.

I'm also helped so much by the spirit of human kindness, which follows me everywhere, leading to unexpected things. Both the Fort St John and Dawson Creek Chambers of Commerce invite me to take a few days off to take part in the Chicago Marathon on 22 October for charity. I can't resist. I have to run 20 miles a day – more than I'm used to – to get to Edmonton Airport to catch the plane but I make it, leaving Silver Dream Machine, now nicknamed Charlie, in safekeeping in Edmonton.

The Chicago Marathon is an experience way beyond my imagining, mostly because Bob Collins's family in Oak Park near Chicago are so good to me. His sister and brother-in-law, Nancy and Victor Rodriguez, take me home from the airport to meet his other wonderful sister Patty Agostinelli and husband Rich. They spoil me unbelievably. Nancy treats me to a complete overhaul at the Park Avenue Hair Studio: hair trim, manicure, my first pedicure for years. Beautician Florence Doherty paints my toenails *'Vahoom! go faster red'*.

The miles have been wiped away, says Nancy. Bob Collins rescued my toes from frostbite – and now his sister's polishing the toes he saved.

Two months ago I had exceptional personal news. Eve and Pete are having my first granddaughter. I would have come home instantly to be with Eve. Nothing matters compared to her and the rest of my family. I know how much she loves me but she says her big wish is that I keep going and finish my journey for them all; and I know Eve has the children's other lovely grandmother, Maureen, and Pete and all the family with her and will be fine. I'm in touch with them constantly on the mobile now and I'll be running the marathon tomorrow in my future grandchild's honour.

Next day I'm running alongside 34,000 others. The course is along the lake-front, through downtown and fifteen different neighbourhoods including the Chinese and Hispanic communities. I have such fun, coming 15th in my age category thanks to the 'go faster' nail polish.

I've left the cart with Fred and Susie Grafton in Edmonton. Fred and his friends have replaced the fragile tent poles with sturdy ribs which turned Charlie's top into something resembling a covered wagon as in days of yore in Canada and America. It will be much stronger for the winter. Also Florin Man, a cancer nurse who works 12-hour shifts in a hospital in Calgary, is here with a BlackBerry. When I met him earlier he said he'd get me information about a mobile phone. Instead he's personally phoned the Head of Rogers Communications Canada to sponsor me a BlackBerry, enabling me to write my book and keep in touch with James better. Tonight, amazingly, he's driven 200 miles to bring it to me.

It's winter again. By the beginning of November blizzards are roaring and it's getting very cold across the Prairies. I buy tough material and have a little tarp made up as the original tent doesn't fit the new ribs. A small upholsterer in Mundare sews the red tarp overnight, using Velcro to secure it to Charlie as it's so light. Velcro was used on my sled in Alaska but that also had straps. One morning during a stiff headwind, I'm proceeding along pulling Charlie when I happen to look back just in time to see the new tarp flying away across the prairies, followed closely by two pairs of my trousers. Charlie is completely open to the elements. I give chase over the frozen wastes and am fortunately able to catch them. Roping the tarp back on, I return to Mundare to get wingnuts put on so it never flies away again. After that it's a brilliant success.

It's Christmas. Charlie has a temporary berth among the old aeroplanes and steam engines in the Western Development Museum at Al Capone's haunt of Moose near the US border. A collecting box is placed in front of him by the local community to collect funds for the Moose Jaw Mammography Unit, while I'm presented with a rather daring 'Santa Suit' by the Moose Lingerie Shop 'Pillow Talk' to wear when I give a talk at a fish restaurant in aid of the local Mammography Unit Campaign.

The fish and chips are delicious and everyone is very friendly. I understand why Al Capone liked Moose Jaw. I spend Christmas quietly with friends, thinking of my family, and on New Year's Eve I'm back on the road under the stars, with the coyotes calling and owls hooting.

It's 2007, a brand new year, but camped by the roadside at night it feels more like 200 years ago and little different from how it's been for hundreds of years. At night the prairie still belongs to its wild creatures and birds. Trucks occasionally pass, lit up like great ships, but I now belong to the secret world of the creatures around me. I've been doing this for so long that it's second nature to sleep by the roadside or in the woods and I wonder if I'll be the same again after I get back home. I don't think so.

On 13 January Lucy Stanway, my darling granddaughter, is born. How I wish I could be with Eve, Pete, Michael and Lucy, but I am carrying them all in my heart as, two days later, on 15 January, I cross the border into the United States. It's a brilliant moment. I want to discover the real America, learn about the little communities and the ways of life along my route through North Dakota, Minnesota, Wisconsin, Illinois, Indiana, Ohio, Pennsylvannia, New Jersey, New York, Maine. And I do. It's *Travels with Charlie* in a new kind of way. I often wonder what John Steinbeck would think of this …

I have excruciating toothache and it's getting worse. I go to a dentist in Minot, a big town in North Dakota, who fixes a cracked filling, but shakes his head and says things aren't good at all. There are holes beneath my crowns.

'Buy a sharp knife and cut your food small,' he says sympathetically. There are severe problems with all my teeth as they've been neglected in Siberia and because I've had a poor diet much of the time. Teeth have never been my strong point. I nearly lost them when I was twelve. The school dentist, Ronnie Hackett, wanted them all out but my grandmother had a fit and sent me to another dentist in Ireland who managed to save them. I had to go to him every Monday for a year, watching the grim work in the reflection of his spectacles.

The Minot dentist gives me the address of a specialist in Minnesota and says I need to make choices and should consider mortgaging my house. The specialist may have to pull out my teeth anyhow.

I'm very gloomy – but fortune and kindness are on my side. Van Larson, inventor of 'Get a Grip Surefoot Ice Cleats', whom I met in Grande Prairie, introduces me to Dr Jay Jorgenson. My first appointment is on 26 February. I have to run 28 miles non-stop through a snowstorm to arrive on time. It's important, as he's giving his time free. The local snow-ploughs enter into the spirit of things, ploughing the forest roads extra times specially for Charlie, and we get there.

Dr Jorgenson is a keen, athletic-looking triathlete – maybe that's why going beyond the odds is second nature to him. He examines my mouth, saying, 'It would be fun to put them right.' The first dentist ever to say this about my mouth.

It's a challenge, he says. He and his team are among the most dedicated people I've encountered. Hour after hour, as I sit there, he removes all the fillings and crowns, one by one, and cures the problems beneath. Sometimes I spend five hours at a time in the dentist chair.

'Rosie,' he says, 'you have a high pain threshold,' but it's Dr Jorgenson and his team who have the endurance. He saves teeth nobody could have saved through his heroic efforts – and also saves me from desperate pain.

Over six months between February and June, free of charge in an unbelievably generous project, he saves 26 of my teeth. All I pay are laboratory costs for which I need to thank a dear friend in UK who sponsored me. The larger the debt for the kindness the more determined I am to succeed in the run.

While the dentistry is going on, I keep on running across America. I stop, park Charlie whenever an appointment is due, make a mark on the map. I get a lift or bus back to Park Rapids to the next dental session before continuing my run. I'll never forget how everybody helped me do this. The whole town of Park Rapids are on side for me, putting me up, inviting me in. Park Rapids can hardly be more different from White Mountain village, but their community spirit touches me and I'll always love this little town. Between appointments through the spring and summer I'm able to continue to run 15–20 miles a day.

By June I'm back in Chicago, as part of my run this time, having run over 2000 miles with Charlie since the Chicago Marathon.

CHAPTER 34

Life Is a Marathon

United States, June 2007

I pulled Charlie triumphantly to Nancy and Victor Rodriguez's Oak Park home on 4 June, overjoyed to be back. I'd run like mad to get there and over the last few miles into Chicago I thought I'd hurt a stomach muscle. Nancy is one of the loveliest people I know. I only had a small niggle, but Nancy wasn't going to allow me to continue without first having it looked at. She arranged for her doctor, Karen Weinstein of West Suburban Medical Center, to examine the problem with my stomach and to give me a complete health check. Even Charlie regularly got a check-up so now it was my turn.

Although Dr Weinstein confirmed that my stomach only had a minor strain, during her health check she had found a lump on my breast and booked an appointment for me to have a mammogram at the River Forest Breast Care Center. The mammogram showed that the lump they'd found was nothing. However, they found a tiny different lump, far too small to have been discovered without the mammogram's help. They arrange a needle biopsy for 12 July. If it is anything, the surgery involved will hopefully be tiny

whereas if it had gone undetected it could be a major problem.

I'm so grateful that I've had such an excellent diagnosis
and I pray it's nothing. Meanwhile I just have to get on with
the run. Yet it's totally poignant to me that the one message
I've wanted to spread throughout the run is to get check-ups
early – which all went back to Clive's illness, which is why I
did the run in the first place: the biggest marathon is life
itself.

Gary, Indiana, torn by violence and poverty, is often, I'm
told, called the 'homicide capital of the USA'. Pulling my
cart, I can't choose to go to places because they're safe or
pretty – the magic and hardship of the journey is that on foot
you have to go through everywhere.

It's said that people in Gary are very dangerous and you
must drive through with locked car doors. Yet I have learnt
that if you go into a place with an open heart – although
always aware of the reality – things will turn out for the best.

I spend three days walking through Gary with Charlie.
I'm relaxed in my favourite sports bra and running shorts,
saying hello to everybody; people are so interested in my run
in spite of all their difficulties. People said to be selling socks
to buy drugs actually try to give me the socks and I have to
give them back. When I buy groceries totalling $21 and give
the young female cashier two $20 bills, she says, 'Don't
worry – I'll put in the dollar.'

People overwhelm me with stories of how their loved
ones have had cancer. Just because there are many other

problems here doesn't mean they suffer any less. I sleep in my tent in the streets, and nobody harms me. It's more than that. I feel friendship and kindness among those for whom fate has not dealt gently. One homeless man asks me for two dollars and when I give it to him, he notices the cancer awareness sign on Charlie and wants to give the money back to me.

'You look a bit thin,' he says. 'I could take you off to a women's shelter. They'll feed you and give you something for yourself too.'

This and Eve's forthcoming wedding put my breast problems into perspective. I've decided to go to Eve's wedding – she had originally hoped to have it after I returned, but the run has lasted so much longer than anyone dreamed. I think how often people go home to gather together for sad reasons – as they did for Clive – and how important it is to gather for such a happy occasion. Eve and Pete have been partners for 17 years and love each other so much.

CHAPTER 35

I Am the Wildlife

United States, July 2007

It's becoming very humid running along Highway 20. I drip enough sweat pulling the cart through Indiana to South Bend to fill Lake Michigan. Everything is soaked by sweat and resoaked by thunderstorms, but it's all worth it.

Just before dark on 4 July, needing a rest, I pull my cart off the highway and fall asleep for five hours, awakening to see dazzling fireworks coming from the city, in symphony with the billions of darting fireflies in the sky around my cart. The moon looks down with a dignified air, a beautiful rainbow encircles it. It seems magical, a portent for a happy day.

At 4am it's time to go. The road is clear, gleaming in the moonlight. Sometimes it's smart to get running before your body realises what you're asking it to do; and once you get going it's too late to curl back into the sleeping bag and you get absorbed by the brand new day that's just starting.

The highlight is being invited to stay with Mike and Joanne Jones when I get to South Bend. Mike is a falconer and takes me to watch the wild peregrine falcons nesting near the top of the high city building, The Tower, in the centre of South Bend. Exceptionally, this year they've produced four chicks. It's such a privilege to go 'peregrine watching' with Mike and his friends this evening. The peregrine falcons are quite at home among the buildings, knowing they are safe here.

Mike Jones works with Carole Riewe who is known as a raptor rehabilitator. They have more than 20 rescued or injured owls, red tail hawks to look after. Carole's life's work is rehabilitating her visitors who have been brought to her injured or found in dangerous situations. She nurses them back to fitness and self-sufficiency and then releases them back into the wild.

All of this is a shining light of good being stronger than ill, both in the human and animal world. One of my favourite books as a child was Gerald Durrell's *My Family and Other Animals*. People *are* animals in the most positive of ways. I never forgot this in Alaska, telling the bears and wolves, 'Please respect the wildlife. I *am* the wildlife, please don't eat me.' I admire the work of Mike and Carole so much. The wildlife deserve and need our protection, but also we humans need the wild birds and creatures if the world is to survive.

I break off my run to fly to Co. Limerick in southern Ireland for Pete and Evie's wedding. It is the best moment of my life. It's a joy to be able to hug them, hold them close, meet my beautiful granddaughter, six-month-old Lucy, and catch up with Evie, Pete, Jim and Mikie, and so many of my family and friends. It's only a very brief visit for a few days and I

don't go back home to the UK. To win that privilege, I first
have to finish my run.

It's the morning of 13 July and I'm in a situation experienced
by many thousands of women: I am waiting to hear the
result of a breast biopsy. Even if I do have cancer, I know I'm
in the best hands at the Goshen Center for Cancer Care
under the care of Dr Laura Morris and her team. The
emphasis is on saving the breast as far as possible, and radio-
therapy is pin accurate to save destroying any extra issue, or
having problems with the radiation. I'm so lucky to have
been treated by her and feel fortunate in having the breast
lump because now I understand how people feel in this position. I am so relieved when she tells me my lump is benign.
The results have come back fast, but even so the waiting has
been agony. The whole experience deepens my resolve to tell
people to please to get themselves checked out. If it had
turned out that I did have cancer the operation on my breast
would not have been too bad as the lump was still small.
Early diagnosis is everything. As Clive would want with all
his brave heart, I am now more determined than ever to
spread the message: *early cancer screening saves lives.*

The next town after Goshen is Shipshewana where an
Amish community live. The Amish people use only horses
and bicycles for transport, but their horses are like those in
trotting races, going faster than most city traffic. Speeding
along after dark, with their carriages all lit up, these animals
appear like phantom or magical horses, straight out of one's
dreams. The Amish philosophy is special. They are shy but

laugh a lot with you if you make friends with them. They are generous and sweet-natured, an honest, hard-working, close-knit community, living a simple, thoughtful life.

My cart has its worn harness and shaft fittings brilliantly mended and reworked by a clever Amish harness-maker called Sue and her companions. I'm jumping around with excitement, and Sue says, 'This horse won't hold still.'

The Amish normally don't allow their photograph to be taken and the fact that Sue allowed me to have her photo taken with me was very special.

Yesterday, I crossed the State Line into Ohio, where the green corn seems to grow taller than the farmhouses, and where gorgeous bright-blue cornflowers line the roadside. Though the corn is so tall, and has held out through the thunderstorms, many of the houses are empty or for sale. A sign of the times perhaps for farmers here. Amish country is behind me. My dream is to make New York by September and be in Iceland for Christmas.

It's the end of July. I'm in Holy Toledo, Ohio, only 541 miles from New York, when thunderstorms wake me at 5am – better than an alarm clock. I put on my fine neon reflective police raincoat and run along Central Avenue. It's as if the skies know that recently I've been writing again about Alaska and the Aurora Borealis, and wish to emulate these in a different way. I run to an extraordinary entertainment of lightning flashes bursting like fireworks just before dawn. The next city is Cleveland, 114 miles away.

CHAPTER 36

Running Against
the Current

United States, August–September 2007

Tomorrow, 26 August, is a red-letter day. It will be very special to meet up with Steven Seaton again who has supported me so very generously right from the start.

I last saw Steven 16 months earlier in the wilds of Alaska after pulling my sled up the frozen Yukon River in temperatures of –62°C. Now, thousands of miles and a world away as I arrive in Cincinnati to meet him, the temperature has soared. The hottest day since 1948. Schools have closed early because of the extreme humidity and heat. Already, far into Pennsylvania, I've left Charlie at Clarion to make a day-and-a-half's trip to Cincinnati to meet Steven. My run is easy compared with many people's lives around here. In early summer a drought spoilt the hay crops. The rains came too late to save it but recently the rain has seldom stopped. There's a lot on the news about people's despair in losing their homes from the flooding: over 4200 people are homeless in Minnesota alone, and a state of emergency has been declared.

The sky is giving me a great many torrential free baths. One night I go to sleep listening to the frogs croaking loudly outside and think, *That's odd, because I'm on a hill*, and open my eyes next morning to find that Charlie is floating and has almost become a boat. I am really so lucky compared with most that my house can be moved around. I feel so sorry for the people who have lost everything.

I'm often running up hills and find myself 'running against the current' as water is hurtling against my legs and rushing down at me as I try to climb up. The only way to stop for breath is to hang onto trees or a handy fence, or you'll just fall back.

I'm feeling close to home now. BBC Radio Five Live produce segments on my progress every few weeks, and it's such fun to be talking to people in Britain already.

In the Marathon des Sables, the first long-distance race I ever did carrying a pack, the organisers told us, 'You run with your feet, but it's with your head you stay the distance.' That's as true as ever to me now. Most of all, you run with your heart, for love of running or for the love of the reason for which you are doing it. The inspiring memory of Clive's courage will always stay with me.

'DON'T SHOOT' says one of my favourite signs on the back of Charlie. The sign really reads 'DON'T SHOOT OWLS, EAGLES, HAWKS AND VULTURES', but 'DON'T SHOOT' is all motorists can make out in their headlights from some way back after dark. The sign is fun and I'm proud of it, as wildlife always needs to be respected. I discuss this with Bill and Mary Fitzsimmons and their grandson Joel, in Roseville, Pennsylvania, as they check me out for visibility before leaving at midnight to continue the run. It's so much easier to run in the cool of night. Earlier they wanted me to spend the night with them, but understood that I needed to get on, so generously fed me, allowing me to sleep a few hours in a comfortable bed. When I tiptoe downstairs a blaze of light overwhelms me as I open the kitchen door. There the family are, still busy on my account. All the clothes I own have been laundered and folded in a neat pile, looking like new. Also the BlackBerry, phone and iPod have all been charged up and I'm set to go

Tonight a full moon and stars look down onto the field snuggled between tall forests. As I climb hill after hill, the sky is clear. Yet there are bundles of eerie mist, visible by moonlight, covering the fields, as if the sky had fallen to earth. There aren't many mosquitoes around now, their place taken by thousands of little moths fluttering in the moonlight.

It's typical of Steven to come thousands of miles to check on me, bring kit and encourage me on the last stage of the run. He arrives looking like a pit pony, with many invaluable items including two new pairs of Saucony shoes. I've been through 39 pairs of shoes so far. Thanks to many friends I've been able to access kit in unlikely or remote spots, but sometimes I've had to remember that the art of 'making do' can be a friend too.

One pair of shoes lasted for 1500 miles in eastern Siberia in the unforgettable summer along the Road of Bones. I cut the shoes open, putting bath sponges and bits of foam I'd managed to get hold of inside to pad them so I could manage the sharp stones. It worked for a while, but then the stones started coming in, so I wrapped the shoes in cloths and wore them like that. I'll never take having new shoes for granted again.

No sounds of traffic any more, just birdsong. I'm running along, thinking how lovely and peaceful it all is, when I nearly jump out of my skin. The first black bear I've seen since Alaska appears, crossing the road right in front of me. I've been warned I'm back in bear country, but never expected this. He pauses at the roadside to sniff some flowers, it seems, before shambling off into the forest. Maybe I should feel flattered he's taken no notice of me.

The leaves are turning crimson and gold. Birds have been migrating and the bear looks sleepy when I spot him again next day. It's getting chilly at night. I find it hard to believe the fourth anniversary of my setting off from home is rapidly approaching. So much has happened.

I believe animals and people everywhere don't just make the journey, they *are* the journey. It's true in Siberia, Alaska, Canada, North Dakota, Minnesota, Wisconsin, Illinois, Indiana, Ohio and the beautiful mountains of Pennsylvania. You never know what will happen next. The most enchanting encounters can end up startling you.

Back in Franklin, I meet Gwen, a sweet-faced lady with pretty grey hair, who says she's 71 although looking younger. She invites me to her home where she runs a little shop selling Shaklee natural food products. Generously she wants to sponsor me with some of these products to help me along the road. While discussing this, I look away to examine one of the products she's recommended. A moment later, I turn back to see Gwen *hanging upside down from her feet like a bat*. She's still talking away as if hanging upside down were completely normal.

Rosie, I think, *you've lost it, you need a doctor. You've had too much sun.*

It turns out she's suspended from a long plank with attachments holding her feet. It's called an inversion table or plank. You lean against it, then your weight turns the plank, with you strapped to it, upside down. She claims it's done wonders for her back and knees. Gwen and her husband Bill are lovely. They drive through the night to collect me off the bus in Pittsburgh at 1.30am on my return from Cincinnati and, after putting me to bed for a few hours, drive me next morning to Clarion, where I've stopped the run for the two days I've been away. I'm happy to be reunited with Charlie who's been beautifully aired and looked after by Homer and Mary Lou Watson who I met along the roadside and who had invited Charlie to stay in their spacious garage. All my clothes have been hung up to air in the garage too.

The Watsons own a family printing business and have made me some fine new cancer awareness signs for the cart and new cards for me to hand out. I constantly gather new friends and supporters as my run progresses, but one particular follower in Pennsylvania takes me completely by surprise ...

On 12 September I'm off to Danville, a pretty town two-thirds of the way through Pennsylvania. It will be fun to get there. Rain has been dripping through my tent and I've lovingly wiped the BlackBerry, praying it will keep working in spite of being a little damp. Tonight I'll sleep in a bed, enjoying the luxury of a bath, thanks to the hospitality of the Pine Barn Inn in Danville.

Charlie is still my home most of the time: it's the only way I can do so many miles effectively and within my budget. It's vital to keep focused and organised, and living in Charlie, I can do watches, as at sea, four hours' running, four hours' sleep, and so on. Buying a new bike computer, and a gift from Stan in State College of a bright rear-light, help enormously with night work. It's so good to be very visible and to be able to keep a track of the mileage more easily.

Then on 22 September I discover I have a stowaway, the latest in a list of characters who've fancied sharing my journey. It's not so hard. You can't lock a tent. The fearless golden forest mice in Siberia used to gnaw their way in and if they found the food was out of reach in a tin, they'd nibble my clothes with relish instead. It got so that they trained me to leave a small amount of oatmeal or buckwheat outside, a good distance away, as rent. More recently, when I parked the cart in a garage before heading off to the dentist, a tiny shrew leapt out and rushed off, almost frightening to death the kind lady who was going to look after Charlie. I'll never know how long he'd been riding with me.

It's a pitch-black moonless night outside; no rustling, no squawking. Even the wind's asleep in this little clearing in the woods, not far from the New Jersey border. If there are forty shades of green in Ireland, there are forty shades of silence in the wild woods. The quiet is profound. It's cold, the chilliest September night so far. Condensation in the tent has half frozen into icy diamonds in the torchlight. You really notice how early autumn comes when you're sleeping in a tent.

It should be total peace yet I've suddenly woken, convinced I'm no longer alone. Then I see it. I'm being watched silently by a snake, comfortably coiled in a fold of my favourite Peter Hutchinson Design Minimus sleeping bag. This snake has great taste. He's slender, 3ft long, with a little flickering tongue, bright eyes, leaf-green skin.

It isn't a dangerous snake – the only dangerous snakes in this area are rattlers – but my heart is thudding anyway. It's such a surprise. Never in four years' circumnavigating the globe through so much wilderness have I even seen a snake, never mind right here in bed with me.

I'm concerned he might have come inside because it's colder than usual for the time of year. It could be a young snake without experience. But he definitely can't stay. I have to get him to leave and return to his habitat in the woods before I pull the cart back on the road or he might slither out when it gets warmer later and be run over by traffic. I think he's read my mind and clearly has no plans to leave. He's looking relaxed, almost tame, but disappears like lightning into the depths of the sleeping bags when I try to catch him. That is a mistake from his point of view, because I'm able to close the top of the bag and have him. I get a box, which yesterday someone filled with vegetables, and empty it, making a little nest with an old T-shirt and some paper napkins. Gently I let him fall from the sleeping bag into the box, shut and tie it firmly, as fast as I can before heading into the woods with the box and my torch.

I stumble over ferns, bushes and deep patches of moss, remembering how I used to go into the woods as a child with my four donkeys, seven pet goats, pet cow and dog. My grandmother encouraged me to write a book about animals who brought me up but even she would have been surprised by the snake. I carry him for a mile in the dark. I build a shelter of sticks and leaves, open the box to release him but he stays put. Local people inform me he's probably a garden snake and when I check again later, he's disappeared into this natural wild garden.

From here I strike out for the New Jersey border, and on towards the Big Apple.

CHAPTER 37

New York, New York

United States, October 2007

Three images will stay with me for ever: my first sight of the Statue of Liberty for 24 years; Ellis Island; and Charlie nearly taking a swim.

It's 3 October. I'm running as fast as I can over a bridge from Newark to Jersey City. As so often, Charlie is too fat to go on the footbridge. Instead he has to be a 'vehicle', even though his only engines are my legs.

I'm wedged in traffic as I often have to be. Giant trucks and general traffic roar like a great pack around me, inches from Charlie's wheels and my shafts. The nice people of Newark say they think the bridge is for pedestrians because it's not an interstate highway, but it might be very dangerous. They've never known any pedestrian brave it, except on that narrow footbridge where even more definitely Charlie can't travel.

My only option is to try the main thoroughfare on foot. Somehow pulling a cart one is caught between the pedestrian and mechanised worlds. It strikes me how misleading the term 'pedestrian' can be. As in Moscow, Minneapolis and Chicago, this crossing promises to be a huge, exacting, difficult adventure in itself. The only thing to do is to try and be careful and go for it. The first miracle is just how kind and patient motorists are. Nobody's angry, perhaps helped by the wonderfully clear signs on my cart, designed by the Goshen Center for Cancer Care, explaining my reasons for running.

I'm hauling up to the brow of the bridge, head down, pulling with all my might, like a dray-horse. At the top, I take a big breath, look up and there, ahead of me, beckoning me on from the distance, is Liberty. My knees go all shaky, as many memories overwhelm me.

Last time I saw Liberty was after another huge, solitary journey, at the end of my solo voyage in a 17ft waterline plywood sailing boat from Wales, UK, to New York in 1983. That voyage took 70 days because of storms and because the boat was so small. It was such a strange experience not to see a human face, tree, or animal for 70 days. I'd run out of food five days before the end of the voyage, and was light-headed, but so joyful that my navigation had been accurate enough by sextants to arrive in New York Harbour after 4526 nautical miles, from Hobb's Point in Pembrokeshire. I was first greeted by some children in a fishing boat who called out, 'Hey there! Are you the sailing Annie Oakley?' before being officially met and welcomed by customs officers who presented me with the flag from their customs' launch. The State of New York and Borough of Staten Island had even given me a document proclaiming 4 October 1983 as 'Rosie Swale Day'!

History is repeating itself. Wrapped in faraway thoughts, I'm startled when two police-cars drive up and stop. I'm worried I'm in trouble for crossing the bridge, but then realise they're cheering and waving. I'm nearly in tears when two of these lovely officers give me a Jersey Police Stripe, to commemorate the fact that my run has taken four years and one day so far.

They escort me royally across a busy intersection after the bridge, giving me directions to Liberty Park Camp Site, close to Liberty itself. On arriving I curl up in my sleeping bag, leaving Charlie's tent back-flap open, and gaze at the Statue of Liberty until I eventually doze off. I think of the past, of the countless thousands of courageous people who left their homes, lining up at Ellis Island for a new life, for freedom's sake.

I'm pleased to have the opportunity in the next few days to act as tourism ambassador for Great Britain, and Wales in particular, while in New York, through a series of interviews arranged by Visit Britain and the Welsh Assembly representative in New York.

I receive a fabulous welcome in Times Square and can hardly believe the warmth of the people who cheer Charlie and me into a special Manhattan Finish, where a photocall has been arranged. I'm always haunted by the fact that I'm running around the world with many promises to keep. It isn't good enough just to achieve my personal goal unless it helps the causes I hold so dear. But what I expect to be a small celebration giving valuable publicity to my causes turns into a huge party, thanks to the efforts of Catrin Brace, Andrew Weir and others.

The whole jam-packed effervescent Square seems to stop in its tracks to cheer Charlie. Crowds and traffic part like the Red Sea to make a path as I sprint in a few moments before 2pm. It's a brilliant, spontaneous celebration belonging to everybody.

Catrin and Andrew crown the moment by symbolically giving me the Welsh Red Dragon and Union Jack to fly with pride. It's very rare for them to fly together and a big lump forms in my throat, knowing I'm running for my country. It's suddenly over, but the glow stays with me. Everyone seems happy I've booked a hotel to ensure a good night's rest. But although they're delighted to have me, and a king-sized bed and hot bath await me, there's nowhere to park Charlie. I'm quickly learning that every inch of space in Manhattan is worth its weight in gold. Car-park managers tell me it would be more than their jobs are worth to take Charlie in. I sympathise: although New Yorkers have big hearts and want to do everything for you, they're curtailed by security rules since 9/11. Any 'vehicle' left in a car-park must have an engine and licence number-plate. I say goodbye to the hotel, arriving among the statues and gracious old trees of Central Park, where many people hang out as it's still only 8pm.

I'm getting very tired and think, 'I'll rest here awhile.' I don't wake up until next morning.

Trees glow golden in early morning sunlight, birds sing, early runners and joggers exercise, and dogs join in the fun. A brand new day has arrived and it hardly seems a moment since yesterday. A policeman comes up as I'm leaving, wishing me luck and Godspeed, signs my notebook and wants to

give me a NYPD police stripe to add to the Jersey City
Police stripe. I'm soon being messaged on my BlackBerry by
the *New York Daily News*. A reader has called the paper,
fearing the policeman has been ticketing me, but I assure
them the police have shown me nothing but kindness.

The newspaper sweeps me away for a follow-up spread in
their pages. I want to set the record straight on how good the
NYPD have been to me. Jane, the kind features writer,
won't hear of my going back to the park and arranges for the
newspaper to store Charlie inside their office, and for them
to sponsor me a night in a gorgeous hotel in Times Square.

It's extraordinary. I'm on the 43rd floor and have a quiet
night, gazing down in wonder at the bright lights of the city
spread below me. But I can't think of myself as Cinderella
for sleeping in Central Park as it's been a beautiful, unforgettable experience. I run up Madison Avenue, where the
entire exquisitely dressed staff of Chanel turn out to greet
me, presenting me with a bottle of Chanel No. 5.

On my way through Harlem, I run through a part of the
city where even rap music has been turned down as everybody is in mourning for two people stabbed by a madman,
not far away from me, earlier today. Further on there are
dozens of police-cars with flashing lights. There's been an
explosion nearby with many people hurt. The Mayor of
New York is there right now, visiting the injured.

I carry on over a bridge going north out of Manhattan
and through the Bronx. Here the rap is deafeningly cheer-
ful, belting out of every doorway and car window. It's
getting dark again so I stop at a small tyre-repair store and
ask the owner if I can park in the forecourt for the night.

He agrees and I sleep very well. Next morning, while running through a poor, run-down area, I dodge a rat dashing across the pavement. Garbage is everywhere. I watch women carry heavy equipment, presumably on their way to early-morning cleaning or factory jobs, but they're patient and smiling despite everything.

People ask, 'Aren't you afraid to run through difficult areas?' It's much worse for the people living there, I reply. A lively old man rushes up to me, shouting, with joy spread over his bony, thoughtful-looking face. 'Hey girl, you're running through the Ghetto, for us!'

I'm appearing on *The Martha Stewart Show*. The show has a warm, homely spirit and is great fun. I find Martha unexpectedly down-to-earth and gritty. She achieves more for my special causes in a few words on her show than I could have possibly done for the whole of the rest of the run. Hairstylist Nicole gently trims my wild fringe while make-up artist Deborah dabs the first powder on my nose for years. They're happy for me to retain the 'natural look'. At least it's better than the 'natural look' I had in Alaska with eyelashes frozen together and icicles in my hair, transforming me into an alien or punk rocker from the North Pole.

I meet the organisers of Paul Newman's Hole in the Wall Gang Camp, which has given pleasure to thousands of desperately ill children. Newman started the camps to give children cooped up in hospital for long stretches for treatment 'a chance to raise a little hell'. The cabins are beautiful roughly hewn wilderness cabins, but behind the scenes are the most intensive medical facilities, which are the reason why children can come on their own. Linda, a director, says, 'We can give children chemotherapy if they need it, oxygen, or anything else they may require. The fun and laughter and chance for a child to be free and happy for a while make the camps one of the most joyful places on earth.'

As always my major mission is raising awareness. I am not able to ask for money simply because it's not practical to collect it along my route. Most money that people do give is through the links on James's wonderful website. If people do hand me small amounts of money I try to give it to a local dignitary or policeman to give to one of the local cancer charities.

I'm now headed for Boston, 137 miles away. I have to get going while the weather is still good. Winter in Iceland lies ahead.

CHAPTER 38

Goodbye Charlie,
Hello Icebird

United States, December 2007

The Amish build superb lightweight aluminium carts and
trailers for their horses and Lila Philbrook, my dear friend
in the Amish centre of Shipshewana, had had the vision of
my having an Amish cart for the last part of the journey as
Charlie is wearing out after thousands of miles. She wouldn't
let me alone until I had one and Steven Seaton kindly agreed
to sponsor it.

On 1 December Lila's sister Miriam and brother-in-law
Dave drove for ten hours in the snow from Shipshewana
with a new cart called ICEBIRD to rendezvous with me on the
North Atlantic Coast, near Belfast in Maine. They arrived in
a blizzard with a beautiful yellow cart perched on their
trailer. I haven't met them before but they have just the same
enthusiasm as Lila herself. It was an exceptional thing to do
to bring it all this way.

The plan was that they would leave the new cart and
take Charlie back to Shipshewana temporarily, eventually
to be sent back to Britain. Icebird appears to combine the
toughness and lightness of the aluminium trailers the
Amish horses pull behind their carriages, with some of

Charlie's greatest features, such as the valuable three-wheel system.

Icebird from the start is a lady, unbelievably cosy, insulated with silver material with an upholstered mattress and neat little matching pockets all the way round in which Lila has put chocolates, spare blankets, socks, hand-cream, a new torch, special energy-giving coffee and a cornucopia of gifts. A little later I'm curled up inside Icebird, very warm and happy even though it's cold outside. Another winter has arrived and it's about −15. Soon I can't resist getting up to try her out and am running under the stars and crescent moon.

'Each day comes bearing its own gifts. Untie the ribbons.' These words are on a card from the local hospice near Machias in Down, East Maine. I awake on 14 December thinking, *I'm going to untie those snowy ribbons*. It's snowing heavily but prettily over the Machias River.

Machias is a Native American word, meaning 'bad little falls', as there are thunderous, dangerous falls nearby. Being tidal, the river is not yet frozen. It's a snowy half-world, between water and ice. I hope to get going fast. My GPS position is N44 43.280. W067 26.689. I've been able to dry my clothes and have a great night's rest at Schoppee Farm, thanks to the hospitality of Julie and David Barker and their family – my first night under a roof for a week. Icebird's marvellous but smaller than even the bed in this room. It's wonderful to have space to check the equipment once more before the effort ahead. If I take the short-cut route over the hills, along a narrow highway, which should be OK for Icebird, it's only 32 miles to Canada.

I want to make it before the storms hit this weekend. I dedicate these last few miles in America to the local hospice, as a small way of saying thank you. I'm pushing onwards with all my might for Greenland and, beyond that, winter in Iceland. I want to learn about the lives of the few people who manage to exist in these harsh places in the harshest seasons. Originally I hoped to be back in Tenby by June 2008, but it's now likely to take several months longer than expected due to difficulties of climate and logistics. It's very easy to put rose-tinted spectacles on your ambitions when you're yearning to get home. The conditions are not nearly as tough as in Siberia or Alaska but it's still going to be a hard, snowy winter.

I have an exciting time in blizzards in Cooper Mountain during these last miles through Maine. It's the 'short-cut' to Canada, It's marvellous to be able to keep going through the snow blowing horizontally and the white-outs; it's impossible to see anything other than the wild ghostly shapes of trees bent over in the storm. But Icebird does very well because she's so light.

I have a grand welcome to Canada from the Canadian Customs Officers, the Royal Canadian Mounted Police and many others, including hundreds of school-kids. We have a spontaneous party. I answer a million questions about my journey, but having lost my voice during the storm, can hardly speak. It's such fun and being in New Brunswick, Canada, is another big step forward. The last miles in the USA are tinged with nostalgia. A special moment was meeting Karen Christie and her wonderful children, Hannah, Christina and Grace. Known personally by me as the Snow Bears.

Thoughts of family are never far away: on 19 December my grandson Michael celebrates his sixth birthday. I call him on my BlackBerry and sing happy birthday. He tells me he loved the Indian spirit stick I sent him. I see my first Canadian East Coast moose on Michael's birthday and name him Michael, hoping he might offer to harness himself up and pull Icebird for a while but no such luck. He disappears into the trees, kicking up an extra snowstorm as he gallops off.

I arrive on Christmas Eve at St John, a fairyland of snow and Christmas lights, with the nearly full moon shining over the harbour. I receive many kind invitations to spend Christmas Day. I'm so grateful, but in the end remain steadfast to my plan. I have a fabulous Christmas under the stars and moon in Icebird. Christmas Eve and Christmas Day see the weather clear and bright. I'm deeply touched by the gifts, warmth and friendliness along the highways in New Brunswick. But the only way to have Christmas with everybody is to stay at home in Icebird. I don't have turkey. I eat spaghetti and cheese but have a great time. Thanks to my BlackBerry I travel the time-zones, talking to family and friends around the globe. By the time the batteries have run down, the day is over. Once running across Cuba a few years ago, I met an old man, a Christian, who told me he thought every day should be Christmas Day, a time for loving and giving.

*　*　*

You can never get used to it, never stop your heart jumping when you're alone at night and hear a noise outside. The sniffing, scratching sounds outside Icebird tonight are most peculiar and eerie. Something is digging frantically. Icebird is buried in the snow. We've been sheltering from the storm. It was a struggle for a long way through the blizzard before we found a place to pull off and be safe. The weather hasn't been too cold, but I couldn't see through the sheets of snow, and it's been a dangerous situation. The snowploughs and truck-drivers are really great, as careful as can be, but it's still tricky; such a relief to pull in at last.

I've lit the little stove; heated the water for a drink and for my precious hot-water bottle. It's wonderful how it toasts my stomach and helps dry my socks in the sleeping bag with me. Also my half-frozen trousers. But I must get out of my cosy den. The noise outside is getting louder. Whatever it is seems to be scratching far too close to Icebird's glorious shiny yellow canvas. I have time to think about this, as the tent zip is frozen solid. It takes a little warm water from the thermos to defrost the zip before I can stick my head out – to gaze at my beautiful visitor.

I'm astonished to see a little coyote, looking so pretty, his thick tawny fur covered in snowflakes. A front paw quickly stops digging an extremely fine hole right beside me. I can't understand why he's so unafraid, so cheeky and bold. He seems, like me, to have been expecting something else. It seems strange to see a coyote on the edge of the little town of Hampton, New Brunswick.

The snowstorm has turned everything into white wilderness. The worst is over, no blowing snow or wind, just snow from sky to land, shutting everything into an extraordinary wild intimacy. I feel lucky to share it with the coyote before he changes his mind about all his digging and scurries out of sight.

I run all next day as the weather clears, thinking of Michael the Moose and the coyote. Soon it's snowing hard again. Every mile counts and I still have so far to go. But there have been worse problems to overcome and I have faith this journey will succeed.

CHAPTER 39

The Most Beautiful Sound in the World

Canada, January 2008

Silence: the most beautiful sound in the world. The storm is over and I have to dig myself out as the snow has mounded up outside. I keep the shovel inside Icebird for this purpose. It's worth it. A crescent moon sits on its end, facing west, as I head off to the east. Each on our own paths. I don't know if the moon has its own dream, but I'm following mine.

It's 4 January and very cold. Yesterday was the fourth highest snowfall in one day in the recorded history of New Brunswick – 52 inches in 24 hours, with high winds and blowing snow. The Canadian Government had to order the mighty snowploughs off the highway after two ended up in the ditch. They could see nothing in the white-out.

I proceed with my head wrapped and bowed against the blast. The four-lane highway is just a white narrow snowy track, with 1% of usual traffic. I'm afraid to stop as it's snowing so heavily and not ploughed. I could get stuck if I rested.

I eventually pull up on one of the turn-offs. It's amazing how lonely and immense everything feels in a blizzard. Icebird could easily end up totally buried. To avoid that happening I keep going. I find a truck parked outside the driver's house. They thoughtfully give me water so I don't have to use my fuel melting snow for drinks. Their son isn't very well. They ask if I need anything else, but all I want is to stay in and keep my eye on Icebird.

I bless my great equipment. I wouldn't exchange the Peter Hutchinson sleeping bags for 600 gold bars, not even if someone carried them all for me. The temperature is now –30 and although the weather is not as severe as Alaska, the landscape is very exposed and windswept, and lorries fling heaps of snow over Icebird and me. When the storm gusts come it's very hard to find a turn-off on the highway where I can seek shelter.

Greenland isn't officially part of my world run but with every mile I run I become more and more caught up with the idea of going there. I am so close and I might not have the opportunity to go there again. I become more and more determined to visit and pay my respects to the world largest island. I would love to explore it a little, walk on a glacier, see the abandoned Viking ruins and meet a few of the people in the Greenland of today. I am fascinated by how they cope in the ferocious isolation of winter.

I do at least have a little time to do this. Icebird needs to be flown to Iceland and because she does not pack down she needs to be trucked half-way across America before she can be flown in a large plane to Iceland. My friends Mel O'Brien and her family have built a giant crate like a huge wooden cocoon to transport her that weights 600lb. I can visit Greenland for a few days and still arrive ahead of Icebird in Iceland.

I say goodbye to Icebird and continue with just my pack and bivvi. Even so, it will be a challenge getting to Greenland. There are no scheduled flights from the North American continent in the winter and no boats because of the sea ice. The only scheduled flights from the US are via Denmark, which would far too expensive.

I am just beginning to think I won't make it when Selina Nylander who has read on the website that I want to go to Greenland contacts Crewgold. They own the only mining company in Greenland and incredibly offer to fly me out with one their mine crews and drop me off in Narsarquag in Southern Greenland. It is absolutely wonderful of them and I am so grateful to Selina. My dream is coming true.

On 12 January I get a call on the satphone to tell me that Gerald Bagnell MD of Nalunaq Goldmine has arranged for me to fly with them on 24 January. Suddenly it's a race to get to the ultimate eastern point of my North American run in Truro. I make it and from there fly to St John's to catch the plane with the miners.

On 23 January there are blizzards and 70–100kmph winds in Newfoundland and Labrador. Early the next day the temperature is –29, plus windchill. My flight on the charter-plane to Greenland, scheduled for 2.30am, has to be cancelled but I am told that the plane might fly later in the evening, weather permitting. I stand by for updates from Steve Noseworthy and his staff at the hangar. I pray that the weather will be good enough tonight.

CHAPTER 40

The World's Largest Island

Greenland, February 2008

Greenland is the world's largest island . Eighty per cent of it is covered in ice and it is famous for having no roads at all between its few towns. I plan to travel on side-trips, by plane if necessary, taking my winter tent with me. I can't wait to meet the locals to try to understand this incredible place.

I particularly want to see the abandoned Viking settlement on the edge of the Kuussuup Glacier in Southern Greenland, which is a five-hour trek from the Narsarsquaq settlement. I set off on 1 February but it is only when it gets dark before I am halfway across the ice that I realize I have left too late. My tent and camp are back at Narsarsuaq, as is the tempting hospitality of the Narsarsuaq Hotel there, an oasis in this tiny settlement. I have to retrace my steps in the moonlight as it is –29 and too cold to sleep out without accommodation. The northern stars are so bright and the moon is shining with a rainbow ring around it. How I would love to stay out here tonight. How I miss Icebird.

The next day I decide to give it another go, as it's my last morning before I fly to Nuuk – I have been here for five days already. I set off early. It's snowing, but the snow makes things much warmer. It's now only −9 and the weather is supposed to clear later. Instead, it snows more and more heavily for hours. It's quite pleasant as the snow is a blanket against the cold, and I have my GPS and know the way. Robert Frost's poem 'The Road Less Travelled' has always been among my favourites. It often strikes me on this run that the real road of life is always in the head and the spirit. It is just as well as I can see nothing. If I look down I can just about make out my snowy feet taking small, careful steps over ancient ridges of wavelets of ice on the glacier. It's an eerie feeling. I keep thinking: *How long has this ice that I'm walking on been there? In these days of global warming, how much longer will it survive?* The mightiest faces of nature can be the most vulnerable. Maybe I'm walking on a time capsule.

Suddenly, right in front of me, up off the edge of the glacier, I see the shadowy, indistinct outlines of the Viking ruins. I've arrived. I can't see further than a few inches, but I am overwhelmed. Alone on the glacier I am moved by the lives of the people who used to live here in this unforgiving climate. It's a hauntingly beautiful experience and one that will stay with me for the rest of my life.

The next day I fly to Nuuk, where I'm generously welcomed by Grace Neilsen of Nuuk Tourism. Nuuk is a vibrant capital city of 15,000 and everyone I meet there is exceptionally good-humoured and resourceful. I only have a day or two there there before I travel on to Kulusuk in East Greenland, my last port of call here. It's a remote place surrounded by pack-ice with a population of only 300. Supplies are only shipped in once a year between October and July and at this time of year it is only accessible by air. The people are welcoming even though their lives are extremely hard. There is some tourism in summer but in winter there are seldom any outside visitors at all. One day I am walking to the village in a blizzard when a nose and a pair of black eyes appear out of nowhere, staring right at me. I jump out of my skin – it's a polar bear. We look at each other but then he disappears as quickly as he came. I dream of the bear for nights and days to follow. Polar bears are so beautiful but can also be extremely dangerous. They are just one of the problems that the people here have to live with every day.

I am humbled by my visit to Greenland. I have only been here for a few days and I have barely scratched the surface of this amazing country and its people. I want to come back here to learn more. My visit here is over as quickly as it began and on the 8 February I fly to Iceland to be reunited with Icebird.

CHAPTER 41

Vikings with Golden Hearts

Iceland, February–March 2008

Icebird has arrived in Iceland. I feel so excited to have her back. It's also amazing to be in the same time-zone as Britain. Icebird and I have a brilliant welcome in Reykjavik. She's wheeled inside the gleaming Loftleider Hotel after we are both invited to stay free of charge.

I'm amongst Thor's wild-giant-covered mountains and volcanoes in Iceland. All's well, but the stormy weather makes the going slow. Each step is serenaded by Nature's mighty orchestra, the thunder of ice breaking up, raging waterfalls just released from winter prison; above all, the howling northeast wind.

I'm camped by the roadside on the way out of town, curled up in Icebird, planning a little sleep and then to get going. I'm so happy. This is my little home parked outside a flower shop, after asking the owner's permission to be there. Today, St Valentine's Day, will be busy for them. Reykjavik is definitely a romantic city, like a northern Paris.

I now have roughly a thousand miles to run before I catch the ferry to Britain from the north-east point of Iceland. The night wind is gusting up. I can hear Icebird's harness shaking. She's impatient to be off to the Arctic coast. It will be a wild run. I can hardly sleep for excitement, so I might as well set off right now.

23 February. Another storm is coming and I have to beat it. I'm lucky Icebird hasn't capsized. The safest thing would be to let go of her but I'd lose her and all my equipment. We're being blown sideways into a deep gully at the bottom of mighty, icy Skardsheidi mountain; the wind is gusting like the Hammer of Thor as it belts us.

Wednesday is typical winter Iceland weather. If I didn't feel the power and hear the roaring and howling, I would think I am in fairyland, because it's so beautiful. These mountains of purest white are wrapped in a thousand images of shining flying snow. I've seen it nowhere else. Being in Iceland in winter is not only the penultimate stage of my run, but also like having run around the world to get to a different planet. No wonder I've worn out about 45 pairs of shoes and boots so far. Rocks are handy for tethering me and Icebird as there are no trees, but this time I can see nothing solid.

The highway runs between the mountain and the sea. Although the conditions are not nearly as hard as in Alaska, I am a little worried that Icebird will end up flying. I just can't hold her, even after righting her. So when the gusts get bad I sit down in my harness like a big lump, so that my body works as an anchor. Presently there's a lull in the storm and I get going again. I'm fortunate the only damage is that Icebird's shafts have got bent and I can straighten them up again.

The next time it happens it's more awkward: I get blown too close to the main part of the highway where trucks are jack-knifing and cars skidding all over the place. A kind driver helps pull Icebird to a solitary building, maybe an electricity substation, the only building for miles. He doesn't think I can make it to the next town, maybe for several days, and so comes back with food for me before disappearing again, as if I'd merely imagined him and his vehicle. That's what people in Iceland are like. I think they're Vikings with golden hearts.

At last the wind drops slightly and this evening I manage to get going again. Icebird's proving strong and resilient. I've also had help and encouragement from people along the way, wherever there *are* people, including weather forecasts all the way from Grace in Greenland, as well as good local updates from organic Icelandic farmers on the fjords. Kjristen and his Swiss wife Dora keep Viking cows, a pure-breed for hundreds of years. Iceland has the hardiest cows on the planet, except perhaps for those in Siberia.

I head off from Borganes and the Hamar golf course and hotel, where the manager won't take any money and arranges for Icebird to be mended as well as doing all my laundry. I'm treated like a film-star instead of a cold, wet, weary hooligan. I even have a volcanic tub soak: you lie in the tub, open to the stars and snowy surroundings, and still feel warm in the glorious heated water. I love Iceland. Borganes is also the first place with food shops, after ten days of slow going in the wilds. Next 'landfall' will be Akureyri, 150 miles away.

The weekend forecast on my BlackBerry says the weather will be fairly bad. Storm-force winds from northeast are heading our way. I still have errands to do. The battle of the day is won or lost according to preparation before one sets off. I have to heat water for my hot-water bottle. It's great when I discover how good it is to keep two clean new Colman fuel bottles to use as hot-water bottles for my feet. Unlike traditional rubber hot-water bottles, these are exactly the right size to pop into my shoes or boots, or pull over my socks for a little while to warm the footwear before setting off. It's an exquisite sensation to put on warm socks – total decadence. The weather isn't so cold out of the wind, but the wind chill is nasty. My toes have been playing up a bit and I must be careful.

1 March. There have been storms over the last weeks picking buses off the highway like feathers. The coldest are the northeast storms straight from the North Pole across the Arctic Sea. It is forbidden by law to go into the interior of Iceland in winter as the roads are all closed and it's very dangerous. One tyre mark or footmark can stay on the delicate terrain for years.

Today instead the sun has decided to shine with all its heart. Crystal mountains, snowy wild landscape, and frozen waterfalls like chandeliers in an ice palace, sparkle as the sun rises. Even the thick-frosted manes and tails of the tough little Icelandic horses become a fantasy pink, then scarlet before turning all shades of gold. I look out at this sublime world just after dawn, drinking coffee.

The colours seem to have more strength and power, like the wind. Everything in Iceland is magnified 100 times. As I get ready, the horses living in great herds in north Iceland, the only animals hardy enough to be out in the fields, gallop up merrily to inspect me, as has become their habit, snorting like little warhorses. They definitely look golden or even pink in this light. Even their whiskers and forelocks gleam as they are icy. They could be from legend. Perhaps I'm running through one of those Icelandic sagas for real. If it's to have a happy ending, I must keep going.

CHAPTER 42

Thor's Hammer and Thorgeir's Teabags

Iceland—The Faroes, March—June 2008

I'm just 198km from Akureyri, leaving approximately 500km of Iceland left to run. Depending on whether I can make a detour via the interior, I may be able to make the first boat to Scotland in the spring. The next town is Blonduos 50km away. This distance could take me one or two days or a week. Two fierce storms are forecast in the next few days, so the sunny weather won't last. Everything here depends on taking advantage of the breaks. I feel greatly cheered as I set off as I've just had another flying visit from Geoff and Inna, who've rented a car, driven over the exposed Voltavorduheidi mountain and met me on the road, bringing badly needed equipment, like my 44th pair of Saucony shoes, heatpads and other treasures. They can't stay longer: they have to return over the mountain to Reykjavik in their small non-four-wheel-drive vehicle, as it would be too dangerous after nightfall.

I feel much stronger and more energetic since I've been using Nancy Rodriguez's tips on how to eat well during the long distances between shops. Nancy started her famous company Food Marketing Support Services at her kitchen table at their home Oak Park, Illinois, in 1985 while her three children were young. Since then it has become renowned internationally, advising major food manufacturers on nutrition and the development of their products – but nobody has been more grateful for her essential nutritionally guidance than one lonely adventurer and runner in the wilds.

Her advice includes buying cold-pressed olive oil. One bottle lasts for ages. It isn't heavy. You only need a little each day, but it's so good for health. I also follow Nancy's philosophy of buying whole-wheat pasta with Omega 3 in its ingredients. Plus I have fresh ginger and garlic, compact to store. I protect the garlic from freezing by popping it into my sock, but have to remember which sock, or running could become painful. I often add herbs and dried greens to the spaghetti, instead of just synthetic-flavour cubes as a basis. I can store plenty of this. I also like keeping oats, honey and dried fish. Though it's simple, this food is easy to cook. I eat everything else too if I'm near shops, but healthy food pays in 'engine power' and I feel great on it.

8 March. I'm excited that I'm getting so close to Greenwich. Icebird is doing brilliantly. She got hit by a flying pumice rock yesterday. The canvas was slightly torn but is fine. She just needs a little patch, like sticking plaster on a graze.

I arrive in Blonduos after one of the worst gales so far. Driving snow has turned to deluges of rain, with flooding on the town's bridge. I wade up to the knees, the wet quickly freezes and I arrive at the school with feet encased in ice, like

Cinderella, except I want to lose these glass slippers. The kindly staff quickly sort me out with hot food and radiators for my socks. They, and the seismic scientist Josef Holmjarn, who stopped his car the day before and gave me food, exemplify the kindness of Icelanders. Feeling refreshed, I go on my way, sheltering for the night on the leeward side of the mountains, perched behind one of the peaks, just out of the wind, as I have observed native horses doing.

Today everything looks much better. The sky is clearer, the wind has eased and I'm on my way to Akureyri where I arrive on 15 March. It's a magical city on the N66 latitude. Along the Arctic north coast whales leap and own the place; a few daring polar bears ride the ice-floes all the way from the North Pole. Icebird, in league with the wild gales, is longing to fly, but our progress is slower than expected as I've had a touch of frostbite in the old injury. The toe is alright now. I'm grateful to the Alaska National Guard medic who taught me how to deal with frostbite if it ever returned. I have to be careful to keep it from getting cold and check it frequently. I can't wait to go dancing on all ten toes when I set foot in Scotland.

22 March. I have to cross a big mountain pass before the high wind sweeps back in. Way back, when I ran across the Icelandic lava desert for *Runner's World*, I was amused to learn that Icelandic mountaineers call it 'doing an Elvis', when your legs shake uncontrollably in fear. It's just as true now. The high mountain passes are dangerous because even in a land like this where weather forecasts are vital, condi-

tions can suddenly change. The people tell you with pride mixed with misgiving, 'In Iceland, anything can happen.' On Thursday there's blinding snow.

A local policewoman, on her way to help a rescue vehicle that's assisting motorists stranded on the mountain pass, says the weather will get much worse before improving after midnight. The pass is now closed. The fact that Icelandic motorists, accustomed to winter driving conditions, need help is reason enough. Everything turns out OK and a policeman returns to check on me and congratulates me for sheltering safely tied to a rock, until the storm is over. Fortunately, he says, no-one has been injured.

By next morning the pass has reopened. Traffic bounces by on giant balloon tyres 'floating' on snow. The icy sun emerges and the exquisite white mountains are reflected in the Eyjafjordur fiord. Wild ducks swim in half-frozen inlets. Some reflections make it look as if they're actually swimming among the mountain peaks. Nature pretends the storm hasn't happened – you can almost believe it. I get halfway up the mountain when the wind picks up again, but Icebird copes because I have loaded her with a few heavy stones as ballast.

I think the 'cold world' is the world's oldest commonwealth. From the land of the Eskimos to that of the Vikings, the law is the same. Get going while the going's good.

By 31 March I've reached Myvatn. Fierce blowing snow flies around the immense ash cone crater of Hverfall. All around and beneath it, a white icy-cold desert is interspersed with mesmerising shapes and lumps of lava sticking up from the deep snow. The latter look like a beautiful lost race of people whose secrets will never be told, though they're razor-sharp and very real. There are many eerie pseudo-craters, some on the islands on Lake Myvatn beside Hverfall, created by steam when water and boiling lava met. Mighty Krafla, one of the kings of Icelandic volcanoes, lies slightly north of the lake. It's all part of a geothermal area where the earth's molten interior is only a few miles from the crust.

At 1000m beneath the snow-covered lava field, the temperature is 200°C, and getting hotter with every metre down from there. Yet a few nights ago it was −15°C where I was, and back to melting snow-water for drinking, since the streams are still frozen. Even the insulated interior of Icebird is covered with ice. There are tasty lumps of frozen bread for breakfast. My cuisine has all the delights of being prepared inside a freezer.

One recent morning my eyelashes froze together again, as they used to do in Siberia and Alaska, but it was probably laziness that made it hard for me to open my eyes. During the stormy ten days and nights in the open between Akureyri and Lake Myvatn, I dream of lovely things like a hot shower, but most of all I want to recharge my batteries so I can talk again to family and friends. Something about being so close to the finish, yet with a challenge still remaining, has made me miss them even more. It will be such a joy to see everybody. I'm not ashamed of the pain of this longing. It's the same for anyone who has been on a big journey.

Asdis Johannesdottir and her husband who own the Sel Hotel in Myvatn come out to the lava field inviting me to stay at the friendly hotel. They insist I remain two days and won't allow me to pay. They do all my laundry, feed me delicious meals and put in a lot of TLC. A nagging cough I've had for a while vanishes as if by magic. Best of all, I'm able to make phone-calls and charge up my batteries. Another hero of Iceland for me is Thorgeir Gunnarsson, Tourism Chief in Myvatn, who gives me wonderful local information, and helps in so many ways. Nobody should go to the Myvatn region without meeting Thorgeir. He is the Icelandic member of my 'A Team'.

After two peaceful, productive days, I'm well stocked up and bouncing with energy, with only 90 miles to go in Iceland, mostly through open lava field and desert along lonely winter road. I won't come across any more towns until 15 miles from the Icelandic finish. It's stormy again as I leave. White-outs and gales are predicted for the whole week, but Icebird has learnt to 'heave to' beautifully, and we'll be careful. She's shaking hard now, making the Black-Berry jump as I write, but holds true. I'm developing great trust in her. We've already been through so much together.

7 April. In the first few unforgettable days I make it over the first mountain and through the desert. The desert has always cast a spell on wayfarers, pilgrims, warriors, those fleeing from justice or seeking answers, and an ordinary traveller like me. The profound silence at night after a storm is like a prayer and one of the most extraordinary experiences on God's earth. You can hear your heart beating; the thoughts of your whole life and many ideas go through your head.

The roar of the wind begins again, rocking Icebird like a cradle. I almost doze off. Then the roar intensifies. I grab my shoes and get out, I decide to tie Icebird up to rocks or a piece of ice. The alternative is to take off and get going. Yesterday at 3am it was still cold even for the first week in April.

The cabbage I bought in the store in Myvatn is frozen, a big lump I keep bumping into as I get ready, looking crystallised, its vitamins fighting for life. The Arctic light is beginning to return but sometimes this makes no difference. There are many white-outs when you can't tell where land ends and sky begins.

The morning is clear. Like the sound of the wild wind after the desert's silence, the first sight of the giant dunes after the limited visibility is especially beautiful. The dunes look like those in *Lawrence of Arabia*, except made of snow and a pure shining white.

The highway is a friend. Like other desert roads, it's a shipping lane through a solid ocean. As I get going, the blue ice on it gets thicker as the road becomes more treacherous every few kilometres eastwards. It's the only way. Just a step or so off the road, there's deep, soft snow up to my shoulders. Although the morning is bright, the increasing wind means the ice and my feet are tricky to see as snow is blowing up to my knees. The wind is also a friend, westerly in my favour, shoving me along, sometimes frightening, but good at the same time. I dig my toes in as much as I can. You can put your life in the hands of Sure Foot Company's 'Get a Grip' cleats, which you put on your footwear to stop you slipping. Native peoples around the world, such as the Siberians in far north, wear moccasin-like footwear in the cold weather. My interpretation of this is wearing my Saucony trail shoes. They work better than booties for me, as I am never indoors long enough to dry big boots, but can dry the soft shoes in my sleeping bag, taking the insoles out. The cleats or spikes that I wear to prevent myself slipping fit over my shoes well, but I am anxious because my cleats are wearing out fast on the hard ice and with the pressure of hauling along Icebird. My cleats also lost some of their spikes on the earlier desert sections of icy razor-sharp lava. It maddens me that I haven't bought extra pairs. I keep thinking, *the journey is nearly over, winter is nearly over*. What a mistake.

It's always down to equipment. My equipment has been through the wars with me and has saved me. I've never been intrepid; it's my equipment that's intrepid. Now it's down to me. I tread as carefully as I can, slipping twice and actually stopping for breath.

I dive into the cart and start writing a report to my family: 'A lot of time is spent trying not to fall over.' I should never have written it down. Ten minutes later, I crash down and one of the cart's shafts drives into my side and there's a cracking sound. Almost a carbon copy of one of the times I broke my ribs in Alaska.

It isn't too bad. In pain, I lie still, deciding what to do next. The first vehicle of the day comes along and, seeing me lying there, stops. The people help me up, worried about the blood from my cut knuckles, which is really nothing. I say I'm fine, though I use their phone to call my great ally Asdis, to ask if I might borrow her cleats, and if so, can she get them out to me. Alone again, I feel I can cope.

I pull Icebird slowly for another mile, keeping the harness across my stomach instead of my ribs. I feel dizzy, but manage to tug the cart safely off the highway. I think, make or break would be whether I can actually bend to crawl inside the cart. I accomplish it successfully, making me feel victorious, and better.

I'm lighting the primus stove to heat snow-water for a hot-water bottle to place against the sore spots when Thorgeir arrives. In this way the Icelandic people are like Alaskans – they look out for you through thick and thin. He came two days earlier into the desert to find me, bringing Mr Pickwick teabags, dried fish, new socks, all kinds of treats. This time he's come by chance to check on me again and also because a British photographer needs more pictures of me for an article. Instead of photographing me, he takes me to Husavik, where, although it's a weekend, Dr Unnsteinn Juliusson sees me at the Husavik Health Care Centre.

Dr Juliusson is very kind. I trust him like the Alaska National Guard medics, knowing his advice is sound. He's aware I need to get to the finish safely. I've broken at least two ribs near the spinal column, though it isn't dangerous because it's not near a lung. I've also damaged the front ribs, but not seriously. It would be much worse, as far as my run is concerned, if I'd broken an ankle. The only problem is that Dr Juliusson says setting it would make the injury less likely to heal quickly and could cause more damage.

I don't want to run through pain or be hobbling on arrival in Britain. It will be 4–6 weeks until everything has healed properly but, if I use pain as a guide, he says I'll be able to set off with Icebird in about two weeks. At least it means that Icebird herself can be mended. Her shafts and harness require better repairs than my faithful duct tape provides. Icebird has a short rest, while I've been delightfully coerced by Asdis to spend the first few nights fast-forwarding the healing of the ribs in the gorgeous Sel-Hotel. After that I'll go to live in Icebird beside Lake Myvatn, because I want to stay hardy. In any case, Icebird is such a dear little home and we're in this whole epic Icelandic adventure together.

When I'm better, my friends will take Icebird and me back to the spot where I fell. It's only 60 miles from there to the east coast. While my ribs heal, the harness is sent to a professional saddler in Akureyri, and I arrange for the 66 North Sports Shop in Akureyri to send me two pairs of new cleats. One of these is to replace the pair I borrowed from Asdis because in northeast Iceland there's no sign of a melt-down. The year seems to be going backwards into winter.

Billions of sparkling frosty stars shine all over the ground, trying to outdo those in the sky. It's 3am on 19 April, and still several degrees below zero. I have to wrap up and keep looking out, because it's a magical time. The Arctic spring light is a promise that the cold cannot break. A nearly full moon has a halo that's not round but a dazzling little cloud flaring out on all sides. It looks especially enchanting as the sky is already turning a royal blue. It will be dawn by 4am. Best of all are these early morning 'finishing parties'. They really only began a day or so ago. One of the greatest privileges on earth is to be there when the geese, ducks and others arrive at Myvatn, at the end of their thousands of miles' migration. It's so moving and inspiring. I'm lying by myself in the empty car-park in my fine little home nursing my ribs, when suddenly there's a loud quacking and beating of wings, and the dawn sky is full of birds – a scene I'll never forget.

There have been more and more birds arriving. The latest is the red-wing thrush. He's hopped onto Icebird's roof a few times, but mostly perches nearby above a lamp post, singing his heart out. Apparently the red wing sings to reclaim his territory. The top of the lamp-post is quite a good spot, not far from the store, with its outdoor cafeteria in the summer, where he can dine for free.

In a few days I shall be starting again. The nurse gave me painkillers in case of problems, but I should be fine. It's sensible to go now, to keep my legs and the rest of me fit and because of the brilliant way the harness was mended, I can pull Icebird without putting a strain on the ribs. I want the running to be a way of praying, of saying thank you to God and to life, and to all the people who've helped me, to the brave voyaging birds and animals, and the land itself around the sweep of the amazing world.

By 26 April I've had time to consider my plan and have decided to set off next Wednesday from the Sel Hotel. I'm not going to be *taken* back to where I broke my ribs: I'm going to *run* back to where I fell and then keep on going. It's only an extra 50 miles and shouldn't take long. The desert's spell is still in my head. I have to see what lies beneath those gleaming white dunes as the melt starts. It's a sensible plan too: I can run for a few days and be fitter by the time I reach a big mountain pass that lies ahead before the coast. Because of storms, it's necessary to run quickly over this pass. There can be ice and blowing snow here until the end of May.

7 May. I've completed the extra 50 miles, and am thrilled. I recently passed the place where I fell. The ribs are history. The endless messages of support I've received have been heartwarming. I'm going to celebrate by stopping here to eat my special 'Gunnarsson Pasta with Cream' – quite a change from 'Spaghetti à la Rosie with Grit'. The Myvatn people still worry about me, bringing me gifts. I can only wear the harness strap on one shoulder as my bad side is still too weak. I keep stopping for breath; the Namafjall mountain, two miles north of Myvatn, is a steep climb. It doesn't matter that I'm slow, because my surroundings are awe-inspiring and a joy to see.

Namafjall is golden-brown. It is part of Myvatn's most beautiful, eerie geothermal area. Steam belches from thousands of holes and vents on the mountain. Famous for its warm nature baths, it's also on an ancient wonderland of survival that has always made a difference to the hard life around here. Locals still cook bread in the steam. You just dig a little hole, put in the dough, with a stone as lid, and let it steam for 24 hours – very tasty. They also plant potatoes in cooler places and can do so long before the icy fields away from the area unfreeze. It's astonishing that potatoes can grow on this moonscape.

My true love began the other side of the mountain. There's a feeling of privacy with nature here in the lava fields that nothing can surpass. Silence when I was last here has been exchanged for the most beautiful sounds and sights. Greylag geese and whooper swans are lazily enjoying the melt-water, nibbling the first green shoots, building up their strength, while their nesting sites defrost. Attractive little snow buntings – the only Icelandic songbirds that stay here year round – remind me of the stormy petrels that followed my boat when I was at sea. The Icelanders' name for them is 'He who laughs at the sun'.

Iceland has a different season several times a day in May. Yesterday, I had shorts on for the first time this year. I washed in the sublime melt-water, bursting in a crazy, happy way from the ice, and already warmed by the sun. There was still some ice in it, but it felt delicious for a few minutes. Suddenly, the sun on the water yielded to black clouds. Shortly afterwards the wind came in with a roaring blast and was pretty stiff by evening. I had to stop once or twice. The weather had improved by 11pm and it was still dusk. A pale sky became full of stars as light finally disappeared. I had a lovely night run and am delighted I can now wear my harness straps on both shoulders once more.

10 May. Outside it's a blizzard. The storm from the east is icy. It can't shift us, because Icebird is safely getting buried in the snow. So much for 'first green shoots'. The birds are in hiding, just like me, puffing out their feathers so they look like round balls. If there isn't shelter, they sit still and let themselves get covered in snow which is good insulation,

useful for trapping the air between the puffed feathers. Icebird does much the same, and I'm snug inside.

By 6am on 23 May, I've made it over the mountain to Seydisfjordur, before descending to sea level and warmer temperatures. I take one last look at the pristine, gleaming winter landscape that I have both feared and grown to love so much, and then descend to where the dramatic mountains sweep down to the sea in the fjord; everything is sparkling. Black clouds, looking like the breath of a giant who's run out of puff, have golden edges.

Here the sun is running the world, stealing the show. The little town is still sleeping. It has a pale-blue painted church, pretty houses and plenty of fishing boats. There's a fine orange life-saving vessel on a slip, just like the RNLI back home. It seems like a dream that 10km ago I was on a high mountain pass between Egilsstadir and Seydisfjordur, with nothing but deep snow as far as the eye could see. It was snowing quite hard at the top, and the olive oil in Icebird's larder had frozen during the night.

I've arrived with days to spare. I'm booked on the ferry to the Faroes from Seydisfjordur on 28 May. From there, Icebird and I take the first boat to Scotland, leaving the Faroes on 16 June, arriving at Scrabster, Scotland on 18 June at 5am. It means something special to arrive by sea with my Icebird.

Meanwhile Icebird and I arrive in the Faroe Islands at 11am on 29 May, receiving a friendly welcome after a 17-hour voyage on board M/F *Norrona*. I spend hours looking at the sea, reflecting on my journey so far. It's beginning to be hard for me to eat or sleep because of the excitement. I feel at the end of something and also at the beginning, and the circle is drawing to a close. Amongst all the colours on this earth, the empty horizon of the sea, like the sand ocean of the desert, can be the most spellbinding sight of all. Suddenly out of the mists the Faroe Islands appear. My first impression is of dramatic cliffs, tops covered with green instead of the snow I'm so used to.

The sun is hidden behind thick cloud, yet the green still seems bright. Little villages lie snugly sheltered in the curves of hills. There are 18 islands; the total population of the Faroes is 480, but it has a big spirit.

I've been invited to give a talk about my round-the-world journey (its world premiere) at the Torshavn Public Library, one of the first events in the Cultural Night which takes place on the first Friday every June. I've also been asked to join a midnight hike. There's nothing like a Faroese summer night when the sun barely disappears over the horizon. You can watch the sun set and rise again three hours later.

We take the ferry to the southernmost island, Suduroy, are picked up by a bus and local guide and taken to the end of the road. The aim is Borgarknappur, a peak on a ridge a little like Mount Snowdon but only 564m high. We arrive too late for sunset but are rewarded with a beautiful sunrise before following the track down and having a lovely breakfast on board the boat back to Thors Harbour.

Tomorrow, 16 June, Icebird and I board the ferry at noon, which will take us via Bergen to Scrabster. I can hardly wait.

CHAPTER 43

Just a Little Run Down Britain

Scotland–England, June–July 2008

I take a big breath – and race up the ramp. Moments later, I'm on British soil for the first time in nearly five years.

It's just after dawn. 5am, 18 June 2008. The ferry from the Faroes has arrived at Scrabster. The Captain put me ahead of the others to leave the boat. I'm hitched to Icebird, wearing my lucky red socks. I'm beyond excitement. I am just so happy and I'm also thinking: *I'm going to put the first footstep, the first footstep, the very first footstep back on shore – after all this time*. It feels like a miracle.

There are tears in my eyes as passengers waiting to board another ferry – who have no idea what an occasion this is for me personally – seem to catch the emotion I'm feeling and become part of it, and they all begin to cheer me on as I run up the long slipway, and go through British Customs.

It's impossible to miss the sight of James and Catherine, holding up a huge banner. I make a dive for their arms, even though I've got the harness on. There's a banner with balloons, saying 'Kitezh loves you' from the Kitezh Community of Children in Russia.

Icebird looks so proud to be piped to the Harbour Master's Office by local Scottish piper John Macrae, amid the skirl of bagpipes; Maria and Adriana representing Kitezh tie bundles of their balloons onto my shafts; Abigail Neal of the BBC whom I last met in Alaska, and Dick Hooper and Catherine Evans from ITV have travelled up from Wales. They are more to me than representatives of the media. They've worried about me for years, sometimes when things seemed hopeless, yet they've kept faith with me.

I love all the fussing and spoiling, which make me feel like the most decadent woman in the world. Everyone wants to know how the toes are after the frostbite so I have to strip off my shoes and socks. The Captain refused to let me stay in the pigeonhole bunk I booked and gave me a cabin with a bath and double bed – but I've been too excited to sleep. I kept thinking of Nancy and the Chicago Marathon, and get out the little pot of pink polish Eve sent me in a loving little care packet to the Faroes – just for this day – and paint my toenails.

As I show my toes off to the world, I'm delighted with the fun of it all, but also I can't help thinking of the actions of Bob Collins and the Alaska National Air Guard. Every person I've met on the world run seems to be here with me today – and the run is far from over. There's still about 800 miles to my front doorstep in Tenby.

Scrabster is part of the magic of the final leg of my run down Britain.

Destiny is blessing me. 18 June is not only the day I've made it back to the UK and the arrival date of the year's first ferry from the Faroes. It is also the birthday of both my children, Eve and James. Eve was born on 18 June 1969 and James on 18 June 1971.

The houses by the shore and along the harbour and all the fishing boats are reflected in the clear water. There's no wind and it's a beautiful early morning, the grey clouds edged with pink light. I leave Icebird in the harbour-master's charge and head off with Catherine and James to their hotel to have a celebration birthday/homecoming full Scottish breakfast, talking non-stop.

Eve can't be here to meet me as she and the family are abroad, but I'm due to see them soon on the way down Britain, and they're here right now in spirit. I can't get over the photos of Eve and the family – how big and beautiful Lucy is and how grown up Michael looks. I wonder whether time is stolen for ever when you're away from those you love or whether it's given back untold when you do see them – I don't know. The edges of time close in. Catherine and James both look magnificent. I can't get over how much both of them in different ways have stoically helped from that first moment when I looked at the map and decided to do the run. It's a paradox because at the same time as feeling they've always been with me in my thoughts, it's such a colossal relief to be here with them. It's so moving and strange to be able to talk face to face.

*   *   *

At 10pm I pull Icebird away from the harbour to start the last leg of the run. I'm full of energy and excitement and race under the stars, pulling my featherweight Icebird. Then I curl up as always by the side of the road. I can't believe I'm in Scotland, dozing and smelling the sweet heather from the moors.

A landmark during my first week in the Highlands is the short detour to the village of Drumbeg to see retired postmistress Non Macleod, whom Clive and I first met on a fishing holiday with Catherine in Drumbeg years ago. Non is loved by everybody, and has been a staunch supporter of my run: she actually phoned me in East Greenland when I was stuck near the icepack close to Kulusuk. Although her body is now frail she has a tough spirit and a gentle Scottish voice full of kindness that stays with you.

An orange half-moon is up at 1.00am on 24 June; there's hardly any night. Amid the hills and lochs I can see gorse and heather, foxgloves and all the fluffy white wild bog flowers. I notice on one side of my camping place something sticking up above the top of the gorse. It's five deer – two with tall antlers. I'm being watched! The deer are silhouetted and I can see them plainly, make out their graceful heads and their ears twitching nervously. I can hardly breathe.

I stay completely still. It's spellbinding to be here.

The plan has always been that the last step of my run will be in Tenby on the flagstone in front of my house, alongside where Nicolas engraved the very first step.

I want to get back to Tenby while the little town is still in the glory of summer; the way I have so often dreamt of it, with all the flowers out and the wide beaches and children digging in the sand and, with a bit of luck, some sunshine too. I think I can make it by the end of August. 'Shall I book your homecoming for the last Bank Holiday of summer, Monday, 25th August?' Ann emails.

The lovely townsfolk of Tenby are going to arrange a welcome so the date is set. I'll have to run 15 miles a day, with seven rest days strung out in between. I should make it without too much difficulty.

It's a marvellous route to start with, along little single-track roads passing Lairg and Drumnadrochit, overlooking Loch Ness. The scenery is glorious and I'm brought back to the mysterious night when I camped beside Loch Ness during training, hoping that I'd see Nessie herself so long ago. From here, I have to take the A82 which is very busy, with only occasional deviations possible, past Fort William and through the dramatic landscape of the Vale of Glencoe to Loch Lomond. That's fine – it's just back to the 24-hour clock. In the same way that I had to run at night on the Yukon as the snow and ice had been packed harder and it was safer; here it's to avoid the traffic.

The top of my right leg, near my hip, has been hurting for a couple of weeks. I think it's a pulled muscle or strain, which is annoying. I've been getting along adequately and my plan has been to wait until I get home to sort it out. There'll be the chance for loads of rest, which is probably what it needs. But quite suddenly it gets a little bit worse.

Rob Reid has been on a journey in Russia organised by Liza Hollingshead, and has learnt of my run. Rob is the founder of the Kintyre Relay Race. He's a long-distance runner who like me didn't start running until in his forties and he's gone from strength to strength. 'Some people have a good cup of tea to wake them up in the mornings,' he'd say. 'Others get up and run!' He's been great and has been in touch on the phone advising me on my best route through Scotland and says he's also planned a guard of honour of local runners to escort me through Glasgow from the Botanical Gardens to George Square on Sunday, 12 July, so we can hand out leaflets about Kitezh to raise some money for them.

The only trouble is that by 9 July my leg is so sore I know I'll have to get it looked at, but there's no time. Undaunted, Rob says he'll arrange for someone from the Athletes' Angels sports physiotherapists, based in Glasgow, to come and treat me on the road. But it doesn't turn out as expected.

The rain is crashing down as I run alongside Loch Lomond on 10 July. The steely grey surface of the water looks as if it's been beaten by nails, and the trees either side of a particularly narrow, bending stretch of the road are swaying and howling under the force of the rain and wind. There's a lot of traffic, and windscreen wipers can't keep up with the deluge, but still drivers courteously try to give me as much room as possible. However, there doesn't seem much chance of anyone coming out to see me, never mind finding a place to stretch me out to look at my injury.

I'm thinking about this, hobbling and trying to run, when a car slows down and hails me. Athlete's Angel Rebecca Joyce and her friend Aengus Shanahan have driven an hour out from Glasgow in the rain to get to me. I now believe that cafes can appear – if you *will* them to be there – just like the Brigadoon spots of Russia. Because, at the actual moment that Rebecca and Aengus arrive, there comes into view a small building with a sign over the door saying Bonnie Brae's Cafe! The rain has stopped, but it's still fairly inhospitable weather.

Rebecca, and Aengus – who is a top fitness instructor, acting in his words as 'physio's roadie' – are amazing. So is Christine, the cafe's manager, who allows Rebecca to set up her treatment table in the cafe storeroom. It's a scene out of *'Allo 'Allo!* Boxes of wine and soft drinks and provisions are all around Rebecca as she works by the dim light in the storeroom. Delivery men keep coming in with boxes of supplies – and almost drop their crates in surprise when they see me prone and respectable – yet practically naked – on a table in the middle of the drinks. I expect René, in his long white apron, to arrive at any moment, but the treatment is brilliant; the leg feels much easier – and the fun and the classy way that Rebecca and Aengus keep working make me laugh so much that I feel better for that alone.

I make it in time to the Botanical Gardens in Glasgow on Sunday at 10.30am and have a great day with the local runners who later show me the route south. My leg, though not entirely better, feels improved. I love the Lowlands of Scotland just as I love the Highlands. As always, it's the people not just the scenery that makes the place; six-year-old Heather Laird and her grandfather Stuart Laird in Lanark help fix a puncture after one inner tube had five holes, and I've run out of spare tubes and patches; and then after climbing the steep hills to get there, a lady runs after me in the street in Moffat to give me a bag of Moffat toffees. Graeme, the best blacksmith in the region, skilfully puts a temporary steel weld onto Icebird's fittings which have cracked, having been damaged during a bad storm in Iceland.

I run hot-foot to Gretna Green, where it's great to see Geoff – there for me as always, and armed as usual with wonderful help (amongst other things, my 52nd and 53rd pair of shoes of the run from Saucony) – to see me through to the end. And then I'm off across the English border.

I do not know if I have changed but the essence of England hasn't changed at all to me. Perhaps it's because I've been away and the edges of time have closed together. The smell of gorse; sunlight on grass; the taste of an English cup of tea: a thousand memories reawakened. After running all the way round the world I'm back in a place where you can go into Boots the Chemist to buy your shampoo.

I run south along the edge of the Lake District. I'm still on my journey with Icebird and living in much the same way as always, mostly stopping wherever I happen to be at the end of a day. I have forgotten how much wildlife there is in Britain. At night I see the shining eyes of foxes, hear owls and watch bats flying. I never need an alarm clock: I'm always woken by the sweet sound of birdsong at 4am, when the birds start their dawn chorus as if they can't wait for the day to start.

By 25 July as I pass through Milnthorpe on the A6, I realise I'm not so far now from Liverpool. I'm longing to see Eve and the family who'll be there to meet me.

CHAPTER 44

The Last Frontier

England–Wales, August 2008

I turn the corner into Ballantyne Place – and Eve is standing there with the sun shining on her hair and a big smile on her face – and with her are Pete, Michael and little nineteen-month-old Lucy.

We stay with Pete's parents Ray and Maureen Stanway in Tuebrook, Liverpool for two days. We've plans to do this, plans to do that, but end up just being happy. There's no question about how the children react to me after not seeing me for a year. It's as if I had only seen them yesterday. We've never been apart. Lucy's favourite colour and mine is pink. She can already say full sentences like *'I want apple juice!'*, and sings Happy Birthday to everybody, whether it's their birthday or not. Michael has recently earned his red belt in karate, and at six years old is proud of me, not because he's been told to be, but because he is – though not nearly as proud as I am of him. We spend a lot of time sitting under the little marquee on the lawn chatting. Later I listen to Eve reading bedtime stories; I love to hear the sound of her voice.

All this gives me so much inspiration over the next three

weeks, which turn out to be more fascinating and convoluted than I could ever have imagined.

The plan is that Eve and the family will see me off on the Mersey Ferry that Sunday before catching their train back to London. I set off to run ahead and they're going to catch me up by taxi.

Suddenly there's a loud cracking sound. I look back and see that Icebird has literally broken in two: the shafts and stem-head fitting are no longer attached to the body of the cart.

All at once this buggy, which has been through 100mph storms near the Arctic Circle in Iceland, is sitting helplessly on the pavement here in Liverpool. She's been thumped up and down, lashed to rocks on the surreal Icelandic moonscape, flung into ravines and onto glaciers, and has somehow survived – until now.

It's wonderful to be rescued by my own family. Within minutes, Eve, Pete, Michael and little Lucy arrive to help. I've always been so proud of Pete. With an hour to go until they have to catch their train to London, he calls his friends in Liverpool on his mobile phone, and soon has everything fixed. Somehow, we pull Icebird, who's like a bird without wings with her broken shafts, to the swish River Bar and Bistro on The Haymarket, owned by Pete's friend Terry Owens.

Icebird is stabled there for the night, while I enjoy more of Ray and Maureen's hospitality. Next morning I return to the Bistro. Engineer Christian Gilhooley takes the morning off work to take Icebird and me to Geoff Truton of Vision Racer, who designs racing car simulators used to train Formula 1 drivers and also repairs rally racing cars. He has state-of-the-art aluminium welding facilities. I owe Christian and Geoff so much for helping at no cost at all. Geoff does a perfect job and Icebird is soon as good as new. It's deliciously ironical that Icebird, built by the Amish who only use horses as transport, has now been prepared for her final stretch of the world run by those who prepare the fastest racing cars on earth.

Later that day I take the 'Ferry 'cross the Mersey'. I'm indebted to the Merseyside Police: from Birkenhead I run along the busy A550 which, though not a motorway, is very dangerous. A police-car draws alongside me. The police officers say they'll have to take Icebird in tow for a mile and give me a ride for my own safety. I'll never forget how when I explain I've run 20,000 miles and *have* to do it on foot – they instead gave me a royal escort, complete with flashing lights.

Next day, 5 August, I run across the Welsh border – the last frontier.

It's raining hard but I don't care as I race across the Blue Bridge over the River Dee at Queensferry. Both Welsh television companies who filmed me at Scrabster are there and people are cheering me on. Mal and Jill, owners of the Bridge Inn, are standing out in the downpour waiting to ask us all in for breakfast. I'm almost wrung out with excitement, being back in the country in which I started my run.

Eric Fromm wrote, 'I swim, I cannot control the stream.' Nothing can prepare me for what happens over the next two weeks.

I'm swept along, swept onwards, by people in a way that is at once a paradox and a miracle to me after the long lonely run. James says there are over 5000 hits a day on the website – it's mostly down to him that people know anything about my run at all. I find it inspiring and deeply moving that as I run through Bala, and then along Cardigan Bay through Aberystwyth, Tanygroes and Aberaeron and on to Cardigan, people are coming out of their homes to say hello, or waving from their doorways; every car is honking; small children are waiting at street corners; drivers are turning around to come to talk to me and encourage me; and my excitement is building, and the joy of it all is increasing the closer to home I get.

I'm not even using my own strength any more – I'm being given the strength by the people willing me forward. The chef and owner at the Emlyn Cafe rushes out in his tall hat and chef's whites to invite me in for breakfast; John Davies – Fastest Milkman in the West – gives me a pinta; the family at a farm at which I call for water have just won a silver cup at the local show with their bonny Welsh Cob mare and her foal, and share the account of their proud moment with me; James Lynch and all the folk at the Fforest Outdoor Store and Cardigan Wildlife Park ask me to an amazing dinner at the Wildlife Park. And Steve Holland, whose genius in designing Hercules and Charlie saw me through some of the toughest parts of the run, drives from Nottingham to see me so I have the privilege of meeting him at long last.

My right leg, which bothered me near Glasgow, is hurting again, but I try to ignore it. Besides, I'm so excited on 17 August as I'm now within 32 miles of Tenby and the suspense is building up in me. Ann has told me that the Mayor of Tenby Sue Lane and Tenby Rotary Club and the Inner Wheel are going to welcome me in Tenby; TROTs Running Club and the Ace cyclists and others are planning to do the last two miles with me; and Patty and Rich Agostinelli are flying from Chicago to be there.

But, there's one final twist of fate: I get up next morning – and can't walk.

CHAPTER 45

Homecoming

Wales, August 2008

The problem is I can't put my weight on my bad leg even for an instant in order to take a step with the other leg. It isn't only that it's suddenly extremely painful – my hip keeps giving way. Not to be beaten – and with gritted teeth – I manage another half a mile.

Huw and Lisa Davies rush out at Cilgerran, insisting I get checked at Withybush Hospital A&E. As Lisa drives me there I feel so sad. I'm thinking of Clive and the last time I went to that hospital. Such a lot has happened because of Clive. I wonder what he'd think of it all. Even though it's Sunday I'm seen almost immediately. Withybush is as brilliant as ever. But the bad news is that I have two stress fractures, one in a dangerous position on the hip.

I'm dumbfounded. I've always had strong bones. The consultants think that the severe fall on the ice last winter that broke some of my ribs may have weakened the hip, so that's why the hard running of the last weeks has brought it on, even though I've already run 20,000 miles without such problems.

I'm devastated. I have to remain in hospital and the doctors say I mustn't walk at all because it would worsen the fractures – and if that happened I might never run again. They put me in Ward 4. The final irony is that I'm not even permitted to walk to the bathroom but have to ring the bell and be taken there in the wheelchair!

They can't take better care of me and one of the big pluses of being in Withybush is that I meet up again with Jane Lewis, a very kind nursing sister who looked after Clive and remembers him well. But I'm going stir crazy.

Next day, already feeling a little better, I steal a Zimmer frame from the Senior Citizens' Ward and start practising walking again – though once I'm discovered, the Zimmer frame is quickly confiscated.

But I'm now extremely anxious. I *have* to get to Tenby for 25 August. Every day I stay in the hospital is one less day in which to cover the 32 miles. Those 32 miles are now more important than all the other miles I've run and everybody's trying to find a way around it.

The first person to visit me is Ann. I shall never be able to repay what she's done for me to make my run possible – even doing my accounts for nearly five years. Just seeing her after all these years is enough to make me feel so much better again. The same is true of the visits from Tracey and Steve, Chas and Carol, and Ward Sister Tessa who come across from Ward 3 to see me, and who's a member of TROT. Everybody is there, rooting for me.

Ann thinks I should drive to Tenby by car and do the 32 miles later on when my legs are better. Alternatively, Radio Ceredigion has been offered a para-Olympic-class racing wheelchair. But I can't bear it. I started out from my home on my own two feet, four and half years ago – and I'm going to end my run on my feet. I'm still determined that it's somehow going to be on the right day too. I should be able to manage one mile an hour.

I'm desperate, but I can't break out of Withybush without the surgeons' permission. I have too much respect for them for that – and it goes against my principles and against the reasons for the run in the first place to disregard medical advice.

It's now the morning of the 20 August and I'm still in hospital when a wonderful thing happens.

The Head Consultant Mr Yaqoob, a distinguished orthopaedic surgeon, comes to my bedside with the other doctors, telling me how his little daughters have been following my run on the TV.

'Please, Mr Yaqoob!' I explain that I nearly died several times during my run, but the reasons I'm doing it are so important that it's been worth keeping going. 'Please, please let me try to continue on foot,' I finish.

Mr Yaqoob is a very great man. He takes the responsibility to waive the decision not to let me use the leg because he knows how much it means to me, and he trusts me to be as careful as I can.

Once he's given the OK, the physios are sent to see me and I'm fitted with crutches. I've never used crutches before and have to practise a bit up and down the ward. I feel like a centipede. Especially, because I still cannot put any weight on the bad leg. But it's *freedom*.

Lisa comes over when I phone her and takes me back to Icebird at Cilgerran. And that evening I'm off again. I still have to live on the road, especially now that time's so short because I need to proceed on a 24-hour clock – start/stop/start … One plan has been to walk without the cart and have it taken ahead a few miles each day, but I soon find it easier to pull it lightly laden than carry a backpack and have this extra weight on my bad leg. It says so much about how easy the Icebird is. I can literally hop into it and have a little rest every time my leg gets too painful.

All along the A478 mountain road across the Presili hills, people get used to the sight of the cart along the verges with the crutches propped up outside it. The crutches are great. It's like having four legs. Part of me does admit that the last few miles are perhaps a test of determination; but in truth I am so full of joy that it gets me through the pain and I don't actually need determination now. I'm just going out of happiness.

More important than my injury is the overwhelming way people are helping and supporting and willing me on. I can feel the power of it. It must be like playing through pain in a soccer match. The support I've had all through my run from the tip of Scotland has been inspiring and exceptional but the closer I get to Tenby, the more people I meet lining the roadside for me cheering. People are rushing out of their pubs, campsites and homes. Hundreds of people. Cars stop and pull ahead of me, the occupants pouring out of them running to say hello and give me a hug; TROT runners who live along my route – Adrian Varney, Brian Williams and

Ann Thomas – keep coming out to check on me. I feel like a film star on crutches!

By the evening of Sunday, 24 August, I'm just two miles from Tenby, at New Hedges.

All my family are there – including Marianne over from Ireland who'd told me before I left on my run, 'I'll be waiting for you at the finish!' She even came out to find me last night – my sister Maude was unable to prevent her doing this as she hadn't been able to wait *any* longer. But I've promised – and it's perhaps the hardest part of the whole run – not to go to Tenby before the official arrival being so kindly planned for me at noon today.

I was so excited I couldn't sleep last night and was up at 6am. Maude and Marianne have brought extra water so I get my green bowl and wash my hair sitting on the edge of Icebird with my bad foot sticking out. I rinse the soap out, then look and see a crowd of well-wishers have gathered even though it's early in the morning. They're laughing at me, but warmly and with affection.

Ann arrives at 10am, so I can slowly walk to Tenby and she can keep the road clear for me so I won't be late.

The TROTs Running Club have all turned out in their blue vests, as well as the Tenby Aces Cycling Club; fire engines have their sirens going and thousands of people are filling the road cheering me in …

… and then, when I turn the corner and see the sea and beautiful Tenby Harbour and enter Tudor Square, there are thousands and thousands more. The square is completely packed. I have never expected a moment like this to happen to me in my lifetime. I never deserved anything like it and I can hardly see for tears.

I am home.

Epilogue

My run around the world started as a journey of loneliness, grief and heartbreak, and the support of a few close friends and family. It began as a message about cancer awareness and a fierce desire to honour Clive and find my way forward again. Somewhere along the way it became a journey about humanity. It showed me that good is stronger than evil, that hope is stronger than despair, that life is more precious than anything else – for everybody: I was so often alone but I found kindness everywhere I went, even from murderers. My run became so interwoven with the lives of everyone I met that it became their journey too. It was as if I was carrying their hopes and dreams with me too. My run became much bigger than me; it became a metaphor for life. It made me see that everything in life is an adventure and a miracle, whether it's running across a glacier or boiling water to make a cup of tea. Life is the greatest, happiest and often toughest adventure of all and I've fallen in love with it all over again.

Acknowledgements

This journey belongs to everybody in the wide world: to those who helped profoundly and did everything for me, and also to those who gave a glass of water or maybe a toot or a friendly wave – and made all the difference too; it also belongs to the thousands of people who encouraged me and followed my run through my son James's epic effort on the website and helped to spread my message about cancer awareness.

Thank you to James, Eve, Pete, Michael, Lucy, John, Mark, Mandy, Marianne and all my family; Bob Collins, Nancy and Victor Rodriguez, Rich and Patty Agostinelli, Kevin and Diana Collins; Ann Rowell who made the impossible possible; Sue Lane Mayor of Tenby, Kath Garner, everyone at Tenby Surgery, Withybush Hospital, TRDT St Clears Running Club, Meryl and David Sharp, Chas and Carol Kingaby, Tracey and Steve Thomas, Anne and Keith Price, Steve Fisher – and every single person in Tenby town; and Catherine Addison, Non Macleod, Steven Seaton, Geoff Hall, Eva Fraser and Marion, Carrie Disney and Richard Tickner, Marijke Engel and Jorg Modow and other close

friends and family who supported me strongly and sponsored me but wish to remain anonymous.

My gratitude for ever to wonderful sponsors, including
Runner's World UK; Liza Hollingshead for her dexterity in
obtaining my Russian visa; Coastal Cottages of
Pembrokeshire; the overseas offices of Allianz Cornhill;
DHL for transporting my equipment; Saucony for their
beautiful running shoes; Terra Nova for my tents; Peter
Hutchinson and his team at PHD Designs for superb
Tempest waterproofs and down clothing and sleeping bags;
Dr Welsby for his great nutritional advice and supplements;
Steve Holland and Giles Dyson, of SJH Projects – the bril-
liant designer and builder of my first two extra tough
carts/sleds; Rosker for my stove; Thirstpoint for my filter
system; and Lila and Rick Philbrook and the marvellous
Amish people of Shipshewana, Indiana who created my last
splendid cart the Icebird. Sir Ranulph Fiennes, for the gift of
one of his ploar expedition harnesses for pulling Hercules.
Thanks also to Fforest Outdoor, Cardigan, my friends at
State College and everybody in South Bend.

Special thanks to my marvellous agent Mandy Little,
Sallyanne Sweeney of Watson Little Ltd; to Susanna Abbott,
Editorial Director at HarperCollins, for driving out to find
me during the last few hundred miles of my journey, and
giving me the chance to write this book; to the great editor
Martin Noble for his faith in my writing, and to everyone
else at HarperCollins.

During the run itself, the memories are indelible. I want
to thank everybody everywhere, even though I cannot name
you all – I have tried to do these acknowledgements over

and over again, and have always ended up with 20 pages – it could be another book! I wish to honour and thank you all so much:

Those involved with the work of the Kitezh Community for Children in Russia; Elena, my first friend in Siberia; the doctors and nurses of the Siberian Railway Hospital and those in the hospital in Irkutsk; Natasha and Fedor; and all the people across Russia and Siberia, often struggling against all the odds to survive and yet who befriended me.

Bob Collins who saved my life and my run in Alaska; Molly, Abby, Alva and Griz; John and Marguerite Earthman; the Nome State Troopers, all the TelAlaska folk, the community in the tiny village of Wales on the Bering Strait and those in all the other isolated roadless Native American communities in the Alaska wilderness.

The fabulous and exceptional Alaska National Air Guard who rescued me when I had frostbite, Major Mike Haller, the medics and Christine Nangle at the National Guard HQ in Anchorage; Colleen Peterson and Dale and Linda Conover who did so much to support and care for me while I was staying in Wasilla recovering, before returning to the Yukon River ice to continue the run.

Will Peterson, Carolyn Craig and family; Dr Adrian Ryan; also Denis Douglas for the loan of his sled; author Jerry Dixon; Sister Dorothy and all the Reverend Sisters of the Diocese of Fairbanks; Al Brawner and many others in Fairbanks and Manley; Karl Bushby, Dimitri Keiffer and Keith Bushby for kindness and for inspiring me; and my friends in Delta Junction, Dot and Tok – and all the way along the Alcan Highway in Alaska and on to Canada.

Florin Man, who is a cancer nurse working long hard shifts, who took it on himself – without me knowing anything about it until afterwards – to phone the Head Office of Rogers of Canada in Calgary and asked them to sponsor me with a BlackBerry to help write my book. I was able write reports all thanks to Florin and Cody Morish of Rogers Canada and construct rough chapters on my tiny screen in the form of amazing emails of sometimes 3,000 words each! The pages would not be here now otherwise!

Fred and Susie Grafton from Onoway who redesigned Charlie's top structure, my friends in Mundare where I managed to buy a tarp and get a new canopy made for it; people all the way through to Watson Lake, Dawson Creek; Fatima and family in Edmonton, and Debbie, Takato and Jim, and all my friends in Saskatoon and Moose Jaw and other places, and the charmingly helpful Canadian and US Customs officers at the border.

Everybody in the heartland of America, especially the finest, kindest dentist on earth, Dr Jay Jorgenson and team in Park Rapids, Minnesota, who sponsored me with work I never could have afforded and painstakingly saved my teeth, after previous dentists I'd seen had said I would lose them all. Poor diet and running out of food in Siberia had affected them.

Dr Karen Weinstein, Nancy's family doctor in Chicago, who gave me a complete physical MOT, and found a lump in my breast; dear Nancy and Patty and family who gave me such special support; Dr Laura Morris at The Goshen Center for Cancer Care in Indiana, who did a biopsy. Everything turned out fine, but I was so grateful for what they did; it reaffirmed my absolute conviction about the importance of early screening.

Lila Philbrook and her friends among the Amish Community in Shipshewana, who later designed and built the Icebird, and Lila's sister, Miriam, and brother-in-law, Dave, who drove half-way across America; to bring it to me.

Thank you also so much to Martha Stewart and producer Charla Riggi who helped raise the profile of early cancer screening, and to Susan Warburg and others, including my sweet friends in State College for their hospitality and for spoiling me; but also I feel profound gratitude to those, some of whom did not wish to tell me their names, who have problems and difficulties and live in inner cities and in places such as Gary. They allowed me to run through their streets and sleep in my little cart without trouble and were so good to me too, often moving me to tears – like the homeless man, who asked for money, and tried to give it back to me when he heard about the reason for the run; and then he said he wanted to take me off to a women's shelter so they'd feed me up, as he thought I was too thin. I shall never, never forget him.

Finally, thank you to the people in Eastern Canada, Russ and Mel O'Brien, Carole Macdonald, Karen Christie and the Snow Bears, Ruth Matheson and all the lovely people here and across Nova Scotia, and marvellous Selina Nylander for getting in touch through James who contacted CrewGold Mining Company who flew me to Greenland; and to the fantastic Grace Nielson of Nuuk Tourism, and others in Greenland.

And to my friend Thorgeir Gunnarsson and all my friends in Iceland; and all those in the Faroe Islands, especially everybody at Torshavn Tourist Office; and the Captain and crew of the ferry to Scotland. At last once more together with my beautiful family, friends and supporters – all the way down Great Britain and back to Tenby, the beginning and end of the circle.

It is overwhelming; I cannot get over it. I will *never* get over all the wonderful people everywhere who are part of my life. I feel deeply privileged and so lucky. I can only thank you again with all my heart.

Further information

To find out more about the charities that Rosie ran for and
how you can help please contact:

The Prostate Cancer Charity
First Floor, Cambridge House
100 Cambridge Grove
London W6 0LE

Tel.: +44 (0)20 8222 7622
Fax: +44 (0)20 8222 7639
Email: info@prostate-cancer.org.uk
Web: www.prostate-cancer.org.uk

Registered charity number: SCO39332

Kitezh Children's Community
Ecologia Youth Trust
The Park
Forres
Morayshire IV36 3TD

Tel./Fax: +44 (0)1309 690995
Email: info@ecologia.org.uk
Web: www.ecologia.org.uk

Registered charity number: SC023976.

You can also find out more information at Rosie's website
www.rosiearoundtheworld.co.uk